I0053628

DENTAL NOTES
CLINICAL AND MANAGEMENT TIPS

A PATH TO A SUCCESSFUL
DENTAL PRACTICE

by

G. BORGES, DDS

© 2021 G. Borges
All rights reserved. Published 2021
21 20 19 18 17   3 4 5 6 7

ISBN 978-0-9906560-1-2
ISBN 978-0-9906560-2-9 (Ebook)

Cover Design: Amy DeLoach and M.C. Borges

Printed in the United States of America

TABLE OF CONTENTS

INTRODUCTION

This book was written with dental students and recent graduates in mind. In it are clinical and management tips gained from having a successful solo, fee-for-service practice for several years. Often in dentistry, there are things that one can do that will make a procedure quicker, such as adopting a routine for preparing a crown and always using sharp burs; or safer, such as enlarging the coronal portion of a canal with Gates Glidden drills before using nickel-titanium rotary files to prevent file separation; or less stressful for the patient, such as placing extraction instruments away from his field of vision. The clinical tips found in these notes present some of these things, actions that one can take to make the workday more productive, successful, in the sense of providing the patient with quality treatment and rewarding.

I recommend some instruments and brands of materials that I found to work very well. However, there are many different instruments and materials available other than the ones mentioned here, some of which work equally well. The important factor in daily practice regarding these is that the material or instrument one utilizes meets its functional requirements, that one become proficient in its use and, finally, that one know when to use it. (The recommendation is simply that and in no way constitutes an endorsement.)

In the post and core section, there are general tips on post use, a section on Flexi-Post and a step-by-step explanation on the use of cast posts. The last two are not commonly used restorative options but, since my experience with them is excellent, I decided to pass it on.

Regarding management tips, while you read these notes, picture a three operatory dental office with one operatory for the hygienist and two for the dentist. There is also a small waiting room, a small front desk area, two bathrooms (one for the patients, one for the staff), a break room and an office for the dentist. The dental chair in each of the operatories faces a one-way vision glass wall. The glass wall faces east so that during the morning, the blinds need to be partially shut because of the sun glare. They are maintained open in the afternoon, which comprises the greater part of the workday. The work hours are from 9:00 am to 6:00 pm with a one-hour paid lunch break for the employees in the middle of the day.

The entire staff of this dental office consists of two dental assistants, one hygienist and one front desk person. There is a cleaning person that comes three times a week, after hours, and does a thorough job of keeping the office clean and neat. The office is one of the corner stores in a busy strip mall with plenty of free parking and is located close to a couple of major highways, making it easily accessible from most parts of the city. The small waiting room also has one-way vision glass walls. It has no TV and is kept organized at all times by the staff. The patient base that is treated in this dental office is fee for service. The office accepts indemnity insurance but no PPO's or HMO's.

It is with such a dental office in mind that the management tips are given. They outline actions one can take for the type of practice described above to run peacefully and productively, and in a way that creates a pleasant environment for everyone involved: employees, patients, and the dentist. Suggestions such as how to educate the patient regarding his condition so that he is better motivated to take care of his teeth, how to keep the hygiene schedule busy, and what to require from the employees, along with what to provide in return, are presented here.

Finally, as in most other information one receives in life, the reader should apply critical thinking when evaluating the recommendations presented here and determine what is useful to his/her particular case.

I hope you enjoy the book!

Chapter 1

CLINICAL TIPS

General Tips

❖ Have a light hand. Apply minimal pressure with your fingers on the teeth and oral structures as you work. After several minutes of pressure, a heavy hand, especially when working on the lower arch, can become uncomfortable to the patient. From the patient's point of view, a light hand is a positive aspect of his dentist's work.

❖ Whenever you must grind a tooth which occludes with the one being treated, inform the patient of this beforehand, and explain why it should be done. A couple of situations in which grinding an opposing tooth might be indicated are a slight extrusion or a sharp centric cusp.

❖ When a patient has reversible pulpitis, it is best if he avoids any additional trauma to the pulp in order to improve the chances of healing. Trauma in this case comes more commonly in the form of repeated exposure to ice cold drinks, an event which stimulates nociceptors in an already inflamed pulp. When nociceptors are stimulated, neurotransmitters are released and there is a biochemical cascade which eventually leads to an intensification of the inflammation.[1] The more often the patient does something that provokes pain, the greater the consequent pulpal irritation and the greater the chances of the reversible pulpitis progressing to irreversible pulpitis. One can explain this to the patient by using the example of a cut on the skin. "Mr. Smith, try to avoid whatever causes pain. Our goal is for the nerve (pulp) to heal and so to avoid RCT. Every time one does something that causes the tooth to hurt, such as drinking ice-cold drinks, it irritates the nerve. If it happens often enough, the nerve can die and then the tooth will need RCT. It is as if one had a cut in the skin. Every time one scratches it, it gets worse and takes longer to heal. Doing

---

1 Abd-Elmeguid A, Yu DC. Dental pulp neurophysiology: part 1. Clinical and diagnostic implications. *J Can Dent Assoc.* 2009 Feb; 75 (1):55-9.

something that makes the tooth hurt is like scratching a cut. The difference is that the nerve in the tooth will reach a point where it will not heal anymore and RCT will be necessary."

❖   Consider having medication for aphtous ulcers, such as Kenalog in Orabase paste, available at each operatory. Occasionally, you will detect one or more aphtous ulcers while doing an exam or performing a routine treatment. At other times, a patient will let you know he has a painful "canker sore" before you start the scheduled treatment. In both situations, after certifying that he is not allergic to it, you can apply the medication to the ulceration in order to alleviate patient discomfort. Also write him a prescription, so that he can continue the treatment at home. Make a notation in the chart regarding the size, location, and length of time the lesion has been present along with the treatment you rendered and the medication you prescribed. If there is no improvement within 2 weeks, refer to an oral surgeon for further evaluation.

Another treatment option for aphtous ulcers is low level laser therapy. It has been shown to provide immediate pain relief and total healing of the lesion within 3 or 4 days.[2]

❖   After the anesthesia has been administered, at the moment when you will start the treatment, make it a habit of asking the patient to inform you if your work (drilling, exploring a canal, luxating a tooth, etc.) is causing him any pain. You can say something like, "If you feel any pain, please let me know. Raise your hand and I will stop immediately." By saying this to the patient, and acting accordingly, you reduce his stress level. You give him a sense of control and at the same time show that you are concerned for his well-being.

❖   An excellent book to have in the dental office to serve as a reference guide regarding the treatment of medically compromised patients:

---

2 Anand V, et al. Low level laser therapy in the treatment of aphthous ulcer. *Indian J Dent Res.* 2013 Mar-Apr; 24(2):267-70. De Souza T, et al. Clinical evaluation of low-level laser treatment for recurring aphthous stomatitis. *Photomed Laser Surg.* 2010 Oct;28 Suppl 2:S85-8

Dental Management of the Medically Compromised Patient, by Donald A. Falace and James W. Little. Elsevier Publishing.

Anesthesia

❖ When administering anesthesia, try to keep the patient from seeing the needle, for even the bravest can feel a little scared when seeing, right next to his face, the sharp object that he believes is about to cause him some pain. A way to accomplish this is to insert the needle in a cotton roll, once the syringe with anesthetic is ready. By hiding the needle thus, when the patient looks, all he sees at the tip of the syringe is the harmless cotton roll. He knows the needle is there but the fact that he does not see it can reduce his fear level. Once the syringe is in the mouth you can touch the cotton roll to the cheek mucosa. It usually will stick to it. If it doesn't, you can hold it in place with the mouth mirror. Then pull your arm back an inch and the needle will be exposed, inside the mouth, without the patient having seen it.

Even with the needle hidden within the cotton roll, try to keep the syringe away from the patient's sight as much as possible.

❖ Deposit anesthetic as you introduce the needle into the tissues and inject the anesthesia very slowly. The slower the anesthesia is administered, the less pain the patient will feel. An area that is particularly sensitive and can be exceedingly painful if the anesthetic is not injected very slowly is the soft tissue buccal to the anterior maxilla (infiltrative anesthesia of maxillary anterior teeth).

❖ Prior to administering anesthesia in the palate, apply pressure with the end of the mirror handle to the soft tissue at the point where the needle will penetrate. After about 5 seconds, shift the instrument to the side a few millimeters, reduce the pressure, and begin moving the instrument at a10 mm amplitude back and forth over the palatal soft tissue, close to the needle. Insert the needle as soon as you reduce the pressure and shift the instrument to the side. Inject the anesthetic very slowly. This technique greatly helps to reduce patient discomfort.

❖   4% Septocaine with epinephrine 1/100,000 (Septodont, Lancaster, PA) provides profound anesthesia. [3]

Time Saving Clinical Tips

❖   Have the operatories set up so that the assistant does not have to leave the room frequently to get the materials and instruments that will be needed during treatment. Have available all impression materials in each operatory: alginate, rubber mixing bowl, mixing spatula, crown impression material, bite registration material, impression guns, etc.

❖   Have one operatory set up for root canal therapy. Keep endodontic files, irrigation syringes, NaOCl, rubber dam supplies, etc., within cabinets or drawers in the room.

❖   Give profound anesthesia that lasts for the duration of the treatment being performed. As a rule, consider always administering two carpules for a mandibular block; 4% Septocaine with epinephrine 1/100,000 (Septodont, Lancaster, PA), as stated previously, works very well. A profound anesthesia fulfills the important requirement of the patient not feeling pain and has the advantage of preventing an interruption midway through the treatment because the tooth is starting to hurt. When this happens, and you must stop to administer more anesthesia, treatment time increases by the several minutes it will take to prepare and administer the anesthesia and wait for it to take effect.

❖   After administering the anesthesia and while you wait for it to take effect:

-    For crown and bridge, the assistant may take the alginate impressions.

---

3 Batista da Silva C, Berto LA, Volpato MC, Ramacciato JC, Motta RH, Ranali J, Groppo FC. Anesthetic efficacy of articaine and lidocaine for incisive/mental nerve block. *J Endod*. 2010 Mar; 36(3):438-41; Meechan JG. The use of the mandibular infiltration anesthetic technique in adults. *J Am Dent Assoc*. 2011 Sep;142 Suppl 3:19S-24S

-    For restorative treatment, choose shade.

-    For an extraction, prepare the instruments in a tray behind the patient. Make ready the post-operative supplies, such as gauze, instruction sheet and ice in a zip lock bag, which will be given to the patient.

-    For an emergency RCT, prepare the materials and instruments to be used. Fill syringes with NaOCl, choose rubber dam clamp, prepare the rubber dam for placement on the tooth, place on the counter the files that are to be used, etc. In the case of a previously scheduled RCT these preparations should be undertaken prior to the patient's arrival.

❖   Use sharp burs when doing a crown preparation and use a new 332 carbide bur per patient (332 carbide burs are excellent for removing amalgam restorations). Sharp burs greatly reduce the time for tooth preparation and the removal of failing restorations.

❖   Try to do as many procedures as you can (if not tiring to the patient) in one visit. Even if it means scheduling a 1 ½ hour, or a 2 hour appointment instead of a 1 hour appointment for that particular set of treatments. This saves much chair time and greatly increases production. It is also beneficial to the patient since it reduces the number of visits and the number of times he has to undergo anesthesia and feel the subsequent numbness after treatment. The time required to clean and set up the room, pass the patient, explain the treatment, administer anesthesia, and wait for it to have an effect can be about 15 minutes. By following the above guideline, your production at the end of the day will have increased while all the following will have decreased: total chair time for that patient; number of visits of the patient to your office; number of times the patient has to feel some discomfort (minimal as it may be); your own work—administering anesthesia, presenting treatment plan of the day to the patient; and finally, your assistant's work—setting up the room, cleaning and sterilizing instruments, passing the patient.

❖   Whenever possible, try to place two composite restorations during a one-hour appointment slot instead of just one composite restoration. If all you do on a given day are composites, and you work eight hours, by the end of the day you will have placed 16 restorations instead of 8. Your income for the day will be doubled, and the number of times the patient has come to your office for treatment will be halved. This, of course, is a general guideline. The time required to place a composite can vary greatly depending on each case. It can take 10 minutes to place a small occlusal restoration, or one hour to place a 4 surface restoration replacing a cusp.

❖   When the hygienist is performing a cleaning on an established patient, in most cases there is no need to wait until he/she finishes in order to do the exam. If you wait until he/she is done, you may, at that moment, be in the middle of a procedure that cannot be interrupted. As a result, his/her patient may end up having to wait until you are free to see him. This is a waste of his time and of the hygienist's time. It can be avoided by your examining the patient before the hygienist finishes, whenever you reach a point in the treatment you are rendering where you can stop for a few minutes. The reason why it is not critical to wait for the hygienist to finish her cleaning when it is an established patient is because his hygiene and oral health should be under control, and you should be able to clearly see his teeth for the exam. If, however, you attempt the exam before the cleaning is completed but are unable to clearly see all surfaces of the teeth due to heavy plaque, then it is better to let the hygienist complete the prophylaxis before you go on with the exam.

❖   Check all dental laboratory work the day it arrives at your office. Make sure it is done according to your instructions. By doing this it will often give you enough time to have the lab make the necessary corrections, if possible, before the day of the try-in or delivery appointment. It entails wasted time and gives the patient a bad impression if only when the patient is on the chair is it detected that a case is not made the way it was requested.

Chapter 2

EXAM

❖   When doing an exam, after collecting all the data and coming to a diagnosis, advise the patient of your findings in a clear but tactful manner. Use the patient's X-rays and show him his teeth and soft tissues with a mouth mirror or digital image to better point out your findings. If there is failing dental treatment, do not be quick to criticize or blame the professional who performed the work.

❖   Write in the chart that you have explained your findings to the patient and shown them to him in his X-rays and in a hand mirror or digital images. For example: "Pt advised of findings, shown caries in X-rays and mirror. Pt advised caries may progress to RCT and eventual tooth loss if left untreated." If he fails to seek treatment and returns with a non-restorable tooth due to caries progression, if necessary, your entry can be used as a reminder to him that he had been advised of this possible consequence of not undergoing treatment.

❖   When a tooth needs to be extracted, especially an anterior tooth, readily mention that there are several forms of replacement. It can be disheartening for the patient to learn that he will lose a tooth, but the knowledge of the available replacement options can lift his spirits up a little.

❖   Look at soft tissues—tongue, mucosa, lips, gingiva. Enter in the chart any abnormalities you find. Refer to an oral surgeon any pathology you are not positive you can adequately treat.

❖   Always note on the chart the condition of the marginal and attached gingiva, whether it is healthy or inflamed, and if inflamed, to what degree.

❖   Look for signs of bruxism and/or clenching: wear facets, bulging masticatory muscles, soreness to touch on masticatory muscles. If any of these signs are present, ask whether the patient feels pain to chewing (muscular) upon waking up. If the patient states he does, this will point to the diagnosis of clenching or bruxism.

❖   If the patient states he clenches at night, even if you do not detect signs such as wear facets and symptoms such as sore masticatory muscles, consider recommending an ONG.

Teeth

❖   Use a sharp explorer to better detect open margins and caries at occlusal grooves and pits.

❖   Dry the teeth with an air jet before examining them.

❖   Explore the grooves in the occlusal surfaces. Be suspicious of a dark spot. Sometimes it may be hard to the touch so that it seems to be a remineralized, inactive carious lesion, when in reality there is a large active caries with softened dentin below. When a hard, dark spot is present, before determining that there is no active caries, look carefully at the BW X-ray for a radiolucency below normal density enamel.

❖   Thoroughly check the distal surface of the most distal tooth in each arch. Often, especially in older patients, there will be caries in these areas.

❖   Incipient caries. If there is incipient caries on an interproximal or other surface, offer the patient the option of attempting remineralization. Explain to the patient: "We can either do a filling or we can try to remineralize the tooth, in which case you may not need a filling."[1] If the patient opts for remineralization, show him how to floss the area and teach caries prevention through diet and behavior changes, such as avoiding: (1) sipping soft drinks or sugared beverages throughout the day, (2) eating and sleeping without brushing teeth, (3) frequent snacking. Recommend a remineralization toothpaste along

----

1 Cury JA, Tenuta LM. Enamel remineralization: controlling the caries disease or treating early caries lesions? *Braz. Oral Res*. vol.23 supl.1 São Paulo, June 2009

with a fluoride mouth rinse.[2] Make clear to the patient that, "There is a chance the remineralization we are attempting may not work and we may end up having to place a filling on this tooth." Emphasize the importance of not missing recall appointments so that the lesion(s) may be monitored.

❖   Darkened coronal tooth structure. If you see a tooth with a dark crown and with no evidence of RCT, check the vitality of the tooth. Perform ice test and percussion test. Look again at the X-ray for abnormalities associated with its root, such as widening of the periodontal ligament (PDL) space. When the coronal tooth structure is significantly darker than the neighboring teeth, there is a high probability that the pulp is necrotic. This happens most often in anterior teeth.

❖   Several chipped or fractured teeth. If you see several chipped or fractured teeth, try to determine the cause. Commonly this is caused by chewing ice. Ask the patient if he chews ice. If he does, show him his fractured teeth while he looks on with a handheld mirror; explain that it is likely his ice chewing habit that is causing the fractures and advise him to stop. If he does not chew ice, try, with his help, to discover if there are any hard foods or candies that he has a habit of chewing or if he has any parafunctional habits such as chewing pens.

❖   Erosions on buccal surface of maxillary anterior teeth. Eroded enamel on the buccal surface of maxillary anterior teeth could be due to sucking on acidic fruits such as lime or lemon. Ask the patient if he has this habit; if he confirms that he does, recommend that he discontinue the habit. Show him the damage done to his teeth while he looks on with a handheld mirror. Explain that if he does not stop, his teeth will become thinner resulting in possible fractures and/or necrotic pulps.

❖   Erosions on palatal surface of maxillary anterior teeth. When the enamel on the palatal surface of maxillary anterior teeth is eroded, a couple of possible causes are frequent vomiting and GERD. If you detect that the patient has a psychological condition that leads to

---

2 Altenburger MJ, et al. Remineralization of artificial interproximal carious lesions using a fluoride mouthrinse. *Am J Dent*. 2007 Dec;20(6):385-9

frequent vomiting, such as bulimia, refer him to the appropriate professional.[3] If he states he suffers from GERD and has not yet consulted a physician regarding this health issue, refer him to a physician.

❖   Non-carious cervical lesions. Often, during an exam, one will detect one or more non-carious cervical lesions (NCCLs). When this occurs, it is important not only to restore the teeth but also to teach the patient about the possible causes of NCCLs. There is a probability these lesions will keep recurring if the possible causes are not addressed.

Studies show that: (1) The use of toothpaste increases the amount of cervical tooth loss in comparison with brushing without toothpaste.[4] (2) Abrasive toothpastes cause more tooth wear than non-abrasive ones.[5] (3) The stiffness of the bristles influences tooth wear, though to a lesser degree than the abrasiveness of the toothpaste. The stiffer the bristle the greater the wear.[6]   (4) Frequent intake of acidic beverages associated with occlusal stresses may cause cervical erosions. A study revealed the presence of NCCLs in patients who were unable to brush their teeth but who drank acidic beverages. The authors noted that the NCCLs occurred in teeth which also had wear facets due to occlusal stress.[7] (5) Engineering analyses demonstrate that stresses produced by occlusal forces concentrate at the cervical areas of teeth.[8] Also, a clinical study revealed a significant association between occlusal trauma and NCCLs.[9] Considering the studies above, one can infer that NCCLs are likely

---

3 Uhlen MM, et al. A. Self-induced vomiting and dental erosion--a clinical study. *BMC Oral Health.* 2014 Jul 29;14:92

4 Dickson W, et al. Effects of cyclic loading and toothbrush abrasion on cervical lesion formation. *Gen Dent.* 2015 Mar-Apr; 63(2):e1-5; Dzakovich J, Oslak R. In vitro reproduction of noncarious cervical lesions. *The J Prosthet Dent* 2008; 100:1-10.

5 Wiegand A, et al. "Impact of toothpaste slurry abrasivity and toothbrush filament stiffness on abrasion of eroded enamel - an in vitro study." *Acta Odontol Scand*, 2008 Aug, 66(4):231-5.

6 Ibid

7 Faye B, et al. Non carious cervical lesions among a non-toothbrushing population with Hansen's disease (leprosy): initial findings. *Quintessence Int.*, 2006 Sep, 37(8):613-9

8 Shetty S, et al. Non Carious Cervical Lesions: Abfraction. *Journal International Oral Health.* 2013 Oct; 5(5): 143–146

9 Brandini D, et al. Clinical evaluation of the association between noncarious cervical lesions and occlusal forces. *J Prosthet Dent.* 2012 Nov; 108(5):298-303

caused by several factors which can act alone or in combination with each other.

First explain to the patient the possible causes of NCCLs and then try to find out if the patient has any of the habits that may lead to them. If he does, encourage the patient to change these habits. You may warn the patient that, "If these lesions keep occurring, the teeth may become sensitive to cold and, if a lesion gets very deep, the nerve may die and the tooth will need a root canal." Recommend to the patient some less-abrasive toothpaste brands (a search in the internet will reveal several lists of common toothpastes and their abrasiveness index).[10] Also, tell him that, after finishing a meal that contained acidic foods, such as tomato sauce, he should rinse with water in order to remove any larger debris and then wait 30 minutes prior to brushing.[11] This will give the saliva a chance to remineralize the enamel that has been softened by the acidic food.[12] If you suspect that the patient grinds or clenches his teeth, recommend an occlusal night guard.

❖   Fractured amalgam restorations. Be wary of fractured amalgam restorations: commonly there is caries below. Usually, the best line of action when coming across a fractured amalgam restoration is to replace the entire filling, instead of doing an amalgam repair or "watching." "Watching" is when one performs no treatment in hope that the condition will improve or, at least, will not worsen. The problem with this approach, in this case, is that it can be difficult to detect the progress of caries below an amalgam restoration. Once an amalgam fractures, bacteria and nutrients can penetrate into the space created and a carious lesion, sometimes hidden from the X-rays by the amalgam itself, may develop.

❖   Fractured resin composite restorations. Fractured composite restorations without signs of underlying caries in the X-ray image, in a patient with optimal hygiene and low caries activity, may be repaired

---

10 http://c2-preview.prosites.com/131248/wy/docs/131248_rdh%20sheet.pdf
11 Attin T, et al. Brushing abrasion of softened and remineralized dentin: an in situ study. *Caries Res.* 2004 Jan-Feb; 38(1):62-6.
12 Humphrey SP, Williamson RT. A review of saliva: Normal composition, flow, and function. *J Prosthet Dent.* 2001 Feb; 85(2):162–9.

instead of replaced. A long-term clinical evaluation study showed this to be a viable treatment option.[13] When deciding whether to replace or repair a resin composite restoration, one must also keep in mind that when replacing a resin composite restoration, because it looks similar to tooth structure, one may inadvertently also remove healthy dentin.

❖   Generalized cervical-buccal caries. Occasionally a patient may present with caries and white demineralization lesions in the cervical-buccal surfaces of several mandibular teeth, often accompanied by caries on maxillary teeth. One of the possible causes for this is the habit of sipping soft drinks (or sports drinks) throughout the day.[14] Sometimes, the patient will even come into the operatory holding a bottle of soda.

When you see these lesions, ask the patient if he has this habit. If he does sip soft drinks throughout the day, teach him that it is harmful and why it is so: "The soda is acidic and demineralizes one's teeth. When one finishes the drink, the saliva normally remineralizes the teeth. But if the soda remains in the mouth for too long, such as when one sips it throughout the day, the saliva does not get a chance to remineralize the teeth and, as a result, these cavities form."[15] Show him the lesions while he looks on with a handheld mirror. Be kind and understanding while you discuss the problem with the patient. Often these patients take medications for mood disorders which reduce the salivary flow. If so, explain to the patient that because he takes a medication that dries his mouth, there is less saliva to counteract the action of the acidic drink and, therefore, he "must be extra careful when drinking soft drinks." Tell him it is okay to have a soda, but it is better not to sip it over a long period of time. Recommend he sip water instead of soft drinks.

13 Gordan V, et al. A long-term evaluation of alternative treatments to replacement of resin-based composite restorations: results of a seven-year study. *J Am Dent Assoc.* 2009 Dec; 140(12):1476-84.
14 Cheng R, et al. Dental erosion and severe tooth decay related to soft drinks: a case report and literature review. *J Zhejiang Univ Sci B.* 2009 May; 10(5): 395–399
15 Dowd FJ. Saliva and dental caries. *Dent Clin North Am.* 1999 Oct; 43(4):579-97.

X-rays

❖   Examine X-rays carefully. Look at the interproximal surfaces, bone and PDL space. Look for tartar, localized or generalized bone loss, caries, internal and/or external root resorption, pulp stones, foreign objects, overhanging restorations, widened PDL space, etc. This is obvious, but under the pressure of a busy day, with patients waiting to be seen, one can become distracted and miss something in the X-ray image. In order to prevent this from occurring, make a mental note that when you are looking at the X-rays nothing else matters but those images you see.

❖   Always have good quality X-rays. The X-ray image must not be blurred. When it is a PA, it must show the whole tooth and a few millimeters of bone beyond the apex. When it is a BW, the interproximal walls of two adjacent teeth should not be superimposed. Teach your office staff to distinguish between a poor quality and a good quality X-ray image so that they will know when to repeat an X-ray. This will save time since you will not have to ask them to retake an X-ray after you have come into the operatory for the exam.

Removable and Fixed Prosthesis

❖   Run the explorer tip along the margins of crowns and fixed partial dentures (FPDs). Feel for overhangs, open margins, and caries. Often, when the crown has an open margin, the tooth structure underneath it will be carious. It can happen in this situation that the caries will not appear in the X-ray, remaining hidden by the crown. By running the explorer along the margins, you will be able to detect whether there is caries underneath the crown.

❖   If the patient has a removable partial denture (RPD), check the condition of the prosthesis such as stability, support, retention, whether there are broken clasps or missing acrylic teeth. Write your findings in the chart.

❖   If the patient has one or more missing teeth that must be replaced, explain to him all the treatment options, their advantages and disadvantages. Compare the cost of the different treatments such as: "The removable partial denture will cost less than the implant," along with comparing its advantages and disadvantages, "The implant supported prosthesis will be more aesthetic, it normally lasts longer, you can chew better with it and you will not have to remove it to sleep, compared to a removable denture." One does not have to mention the exact cost unless the patient asks. The main goal at this point is to explain the advantages and disadvantages of each treatment, cost being one of them.

Continuing with the example of presenting to the patient the treatment options of an RPD and implant supported prosthesis, and adding the option of an FPD, have the assistant bring finished cases that you have ready to be delivered (or cases that you have for the purpose of instructing the patient) of each type of prosthesis. Show them to the patient as you explain each treatment option. For example: as you talk about the RPD you can show him a cast with a metal frame, show the clasps and, on the model, show the prepared occlusal rests. Explain that his teeth will have to be prepared like the teeth on the model. If his case requires a clasp around a premolar, for example, place an instrument such as a spoon excavator over his tooth in the location where the clasp will be. Have him smile and look in the handheld mirror. You can say: "This is more or less what it will look like when you smile." Show him a finished RPD with its acrylic saddles. When you explain about the tooth supported FPD, show him a model with a finished case. Remove the FPD from the model and show him what his teeth will look like once they are prepared.

The purpose of doing all this is to educate the patient so that he can make an informed decision as to which treatment he prefers and so that he is not negatively surprised by any aspect of the treatment he chooses.

Initial Exam

❖   Have the hygienist do a prophylaxis and periodontal charting of every new patient. One of the assistants can help with the charting and can take the full mouth X-rays. When you start your exam, the patient's teeth should be clean and you should have the periodontal chart (six readings on each tooth, degree of mobility, bleeding upon probing) and X-rays at hand.

❖   Make impressions for study models if you plan to do any type of prosthetic treatment, from crowns to complete dentures. Study models allow the practitioner to better visualize the anatomy of the dentition and the surrounding soft tissues. Also, they are an important adjunct in patient education and serve as a legal record. If the case is a complete denture, make impressions of both the present denture and of the edentulous arch.

❖   Enter all your findings in the chart such as: 1) fillings—surfaces, type of material used, condition of margins; 2) crown and FPD—type, age and whether there are open margins; 3) removable prosthesis— type, age, general condition, retention, stability, and support; 4) type of occlusion; 5) extrusions; 6) teeth malpositions; 7) whether there is anterior crowding, etc.

❖   Address the patient's complaint in the initial visit. Sometimes, a new patient who was referred to you may come in wanting a general checkup. You may see he needs extensive treatment but, when asked, has only a minor complaint which he is not too concerned about, such as: "I have a little bit of sensitivity to cold," or "I don't like the color of this restoration" (pointing to an amalgam). The tendency is for one to concentrate on the more pressing treatment, such as periodontal disease and caries, talk about it with the patient during the initial visit, and sometimes forget to mention what one plans to do in order to address the minor complaint. After collecting all the data and doing the exam, explain your findings and present the different treatment options with their advantages and disadvantages. During the presentation, wherever you feel it is more appropriate you can say, "Regarding your sensitivity to cold, this is what we will do…" or, "Regarding this silver filling…"

❖   On the subject of amalgam, there are no studies up to date that show it is harmful to one's health. Therefore, it is incorrect to recommend to a patient that he have his amalgam restorations replaced with resin composite because the former contains mercury. One may, however, replace an amalgam with a resin composite restoration if the patient requests it be done for aesthetic reasons.

❖ Occasionally a patient may come in for an initial exam very concerned about what you see is a mild aesthetic problem. But after looking at the X-rays and doing the oral examination you detect that there is a condition, such as caries, a necrotic pulp or periodontal disease, which must be treated first. When this is the case, explain your findings to the patient. Tell him that the aesthetic concern will be addressed but there is something more urgent that should be treated first. For example: the patient wants to replace amalgams present in lower premolars, or there is a crown with an unaesthetic margin that shows when he smiles, but he also has an asymptomatic necrotic pulp and periapical lesion on a molar. First the tooth with the necrotic pulp must be treated, and then the mild aesthetic concern addressed. If you educate the patient, in this case if you explain to him that a dormant abscess can become symptomatic anytime and cause severe pain and facial swelling, the patient will usually understand and agree with the order of treatment you recommend.

Following the example of the mandibular premolars with amalgam restorations and the molar with a necrotic pulp, if they are in the same quadrant, on the day the core build up/composite restoration is done on the molar that underwent RCT, the amalgam restorations on the premolars can be replaced, under the same anesthesia.

❖ If the patient has periodontal disease, explain in detail what periodontal disease is, its possible consequences such as loss of teeth, and its correlation with health conditions such as diabetes and heart disease.[16] Use photos and drawings to illustrate your points.

❖ If there is a posterior tooth with RCT that is not restored with a crown, it is prudent to warn the patient that the tooth has RCT and may fracture if not crowned (this is especially true in posterior teeth restored with amalgam, though, at present, it is not clear whether a posterior composite restoration with cuspal coverage provides as much fracture

---

16 Abiodun O, et al. Periodontitis and systemic diseases: A literature review. J Indian Soc Periodontol. 2012 Oct-Dec; 16(4): 487–491.

resistance as a crown).[17] Show the patient, in a mirror, which tooth you are talking about. Explain that, depending on how it fractures, the tooth may have to be extracted. Write in the chart what you and the patient said and also that you showed the patient, with the use of a mirror, which tooth you are talking about.

❖   If the patient has extensive caries, try to determine which habit he has that is contributing to this. It could be that he snacks frequently on sweets, or that he drinks coffee with sugar throughout the day, etc. Show the patient the damage to his teeth caused by this habit. Try to educate and motivate your patient. Go over oral hygiene measures. Show the patient how to floss if the hygienist has not already done so. Recommend to the patient a fluoride mouth rinse.

❖   If the patient has extensive restorative treatment, go over oral hygiene and caries preventive measures. As in the case of extensive caries, educate and motivate your patient to take better care of his teeth.

Periodic Exam

❖   Verify if the hygienist has spot probed. If she has not, spot probe and enter the findings in the patient's chart, that is, depth of pocket, whether there is bleeding or not, surface and number of tooth. Warn the patient that he "may feel a little" when you probe.

❖   Use a thin periodontal probe so that it will cause the least amount of discomfort to the patient.

Referring the Patient

For the general dentist, a guideline for referring patients to a specialist is, basically, the level of training and comfort he/she has in doing a certain procedure. One should never "try" an irreversible procedure

---

17 Hansen EK, et al. In vivo fractures of endodontically treated posterior teeth restored with amalgam. Endod Dent Traumatol. 1990 Apr;6(2):49-55. Tikku AP, et al. Are full cast crowns mandatory after endodontic treatment in posterior teeth? *J Conserv Dent.* 2010 Oct-Dec; 13(4): 246–248.

such as periodontal surgery, implant placement or orthodontic tooth movement outside of a school setting, where one is guided and assisted by experienced specialists. Once one obtains enough knowledge and expertise in a certain procedure, to the point where one is comfortable performing it, then one can start to do it in one's private practice. My personal guidelines for referrals:

-      All orthodontic cases

-      Failed molar RCT, that is, molar retreatments

-      Substantial loss of occlusal vertical dimension

-      All crown lengthening surgeries in the aesthetic zone (the visible area seen upon full smile, including the teeth, gingiva, and lips)

-      Refractory periodontitis and periodontitis requiring surgery

-      Implant placement and bone loss around implants

-      Full bony impacted wisdom teeth

-      Certain complete denture cases (see page 132)

Chapter 3

DIAGNOSIS

The great majority of diagnoses one must make in the day to day of a general dentistry practice are straightforward. Occasionally, however, one comes across a case that is not as common and that can be a little more difficult to diagnose. What helps one to be prepared for these unusual cases is to keep well informed by attending CE courses and reading diagnostic case reports in dental journals. Below are two examples of diagnostic challenges and how to approach them.

Cracked Posterior Tooth

If the patient has pain when he chews (usually a sharp pain), which may or may not be accompanied by sensitivity to cold, he may have a cracked tooth. Examine the X-ray image, check vitality and check the occlusion for premature contacts. If the tooth is vital, the X-ray image is within normal limits, and you have ruled out the possibility of a premature contact, consider the possibility of a cracked tooth. This usually occurs in posterior teeth. The four main diagnostic tools at your disposal are:

1) Bite test. When the tooth is cracked, the patient will usually feel pain as he releases the pressure he is applying on the diagnostic tool (a Q-tip works well as the diagnostic tool), that is, when he opens his mouth. Check each cusp separately by putting the Q-tip on top of the selected cusp and having the patient bite down slowly and apply pressure. You can say to him, "Bite down slowly, please, apply a little pressure for a second and then open. If you feel discomfort, let me know if it is when you bite down or when you release the pressure on the Q-tip." Also perform the bite test on the teeth neighboring the one suspected to be cracked.

2) <u>Probing in 1 mm increments around the entire circumference of the tooth</u>. When there is a vertical crack, with time a narrow periodontal pocket will form along the crack line. The probing measurements will abruptly increase as the probe drops into this defect and will abruptly return to normal as you probe beyond it.

3) <u>Transilumination</u>. Turn off the chair light and apply the curing light to the tooth in a buccal-lingual direction. If the tooth is cracked, the light will be partially blocked at the crack line allowing you to clearly see it. If the light is not blocked, try directing it on a mesial-distal direction.

 4) <u>Dye staining</u>. Apply a caries disclosing dye to the tooth. Sometimes it will penetrate the crack making it visible.

When the patient feels pain upon releasing pressure on the Q-tip, the pulp responds normally to vitality tests, the X-ray image is within normal limits and you have transiluminated, probed and dyed the tooth but no crack line has been detected, the next step is to remove any restorations present on the tooth, followed by another round of transilumination and dye application. If, after this, no crack is seen, place a resin composite restoration, relieve the occlusion, and wait a couple of weeks to see if symptoms subside. When the symptoms remain and you are sure the pain is not caused by any other teeth, two of the possible causes for the persistent pain are: (1) a crack that is not visible; (2) low grade irreversible pulpitis. Occasionally, a tooth with irreversible pulpitis may respond normally to thermal testing.[1] At this point the most prudent course of action is to refer to an endodontist for further examination.

After diagnosing a cracked tooth, it is important to educate the patient. As stated in an online article, available from the American Association of Endodontists: "In cases of cracked teeth, the patient should be fully informed that the prognosis is questionable. This is not yet based on research evidence but is based on the principle that it is better to inform

---

1 https://www.aae.org/uploadedfiles/publications_and_research/newsletters/
endodontics_colleagues_for_excellence_newsletter/endodonticdiagnosisfall2013.pdf

and prepare patients for the potential for failure, especially since these fractures tend to grow with time."[2]

At present, in my opinion, the ideal treatment for a restorable cracked tooth is the placement of a crown. A composite restoration does bind the cavity walls together, but a crown caps the whole structure making it impossible for the cavity walls to be separated when the tooth is in function. An alternative to either a crown or grinding the crack line and restoring with resin composite is to place a direct resin composite restoration replacing not only the ground crack line but also the cusps. This is more invasive than the simple resin composite restoration, but it may help prevent the cusps from separating and propagating any invisible crack line which may have remained.

An excellent guide on the detection and treatment of a cracked tooth is the online article mentioned above:

American Association of Endodontists. Endodontics: Colleagues for excellence. "Cracking the cracked tooth code: detection and treatment of various longitudinal root fractures." s2008;(summer):1-7. [updated 2015 Dec 13].[3]

Diffuse Pain on Upper and Lower Arches – What to Do

When an emergency patient presents with diffuse pain and is unsure whether the pain he feels is on the upper or lower arch, do diagnostic tests in both areas, even if it is clear that a certain tooth is a source of discomfort. Rarely, but it can happen, there may also be an ongoing tooth related condition that is symptomatic, in the opposing arch. If this condition goes undetected and only the obvious source of pain is addressed, after the anesthesia is administered the patient may still have some discomfort from the secondary source of pain and he may question the treatment. Obtain X-rays of both arches instead of only the area that you suspect is causing pain. The X-ray will help you in the

---

2 https://www.aae.org/uploadedfiles/publications_and_research/
endodontics_colleagues_for_excellence_newsletter/ecfesum08.pdf
3 Ibid

diagnosis of the secondary source of pain if there is one. Take your time and perform percussion tests, ice tests and, if you feel it is necessary, bite tests on teeth in both upper and lower arches within the area where pain radiates. By making both diagnoses at the same time you will be better able to address the patient's complaint. And by explaining your findings to the patient he will be forewarned of what to expect while the treatment is being performed.

Another possibility in a case of diffuse pain is that a carious tooth to which the patient is pointing as the source of pain is not actually the one causing the discomfort. The culprit being a tooth with irreversible pulpitis in the opposing arch with a condition that is not clearly visible to the patient, such as interproximal caries. The patient may see the obviously carious tooth in the mirror and, since the pain is diffuse, believe it is the cause. The patient's belief that a certain tooth is the cause of the discomfort may throw you off a little, but a thorough diagnostic effort, as described above, will prevent the true source of pain from going undetected.

After doing all the diagnostic tests, if you are still unsure which tooth is causing the pain, a last resort is to anesthetize the "major suspect". If the pain subsides with the anesthesia, then this is likely the offending tooth.

Chapter 4

PRIOR TO STARTING A TREATMENT

Caries Excavation

❖ **Round slow speed burs sizes 6 and 8** – When the cavity is large and there is extensive soft, mushy carious dentin, these burs work better for gross caries removal than do high-speed round diamond burs.

❖ **Round high-speed diamond burs** – In smaller cavities these burs suffice for caries removal. Their different sizes fit well the different cavity sizes allowing for speedy caries removal and, at the same time, a conservative cavity preparation.

❖ **Caries disclosing dyes** - Can be very useful in assisting in caries detection. However, here are some points to keep in mind when using this product. Caries disclosing dyes stain: (1) demineralized dentin whether it contains bacteria (infected) or not (affected);[1] (2) dentin that is close to the pulp more easily than dentin in external walls;[2] (3) the amelo-dentinal junction more easily than the remaining dentin.[3] Also, studies show that tactile sensation is more accurate than the dye alone at determining whether there is caries.[4]

But why use the caries disclosing dye if it has these shortcomings? Here are two reasons: (1) The affected (softened but non-carious) dentin that it stains makes a poor substrate for bonding and should be removed, especially from external walls where a gap may compromise the

---

1 Dorothy McComb, BDS, M.Sc.D., FRCD. Caries-Detector Dyes — How accurate and useful are they? *J. Can. Dent. Assoc.* 2000; 66:195-8
2 Yip HK, Stevenson AG, Beeley JA. The specificity of caries detector dyes in cavity preparation. *Br Dent J.* 1994 Jun 11; 176(11):417-21.
3 Ibid
4 Banerjee A, Kidd EA, Watson TF. In vitro validation of carious dentin removed using different excavation criteria. *Am J Dent.* 2003 Aug;16(4):228-30; Lennon AM, Buchalla W, Rassner B, Becker K, Attin T. Efficiency of 4 caries excavation methods compared. *Oper Dent.* 2006 Sep-Oct; 31(5):551-5.

longevity of the restoration.[5] (2) Due to the small size of the explorer tip in comparison with the size of the cavity, it is impractical to explore all exposed dentin in search of caries. One must, therefore, in addition to feeling dentin hardness with an explorer, rely on its visual examination in order to determine if caries is still present. Normally, one prepares the cavity, looks at the color of the dentin and then checks with the explorer the cavity floors and the areas that one suspects are carious. Sometimes, however, there may be an area of dentin with a normal color that one does not check with the explorer but which is carious or affected. The dye will make these carious and demineralized areas visible.

▪   A way of using the caries disclosing dye: When you finish preparing a large cavity or one that involved an interproximal surface, dab caries disclosing dye over the exposed dentin. Rinse immediately. Generally, one wants to follow the manufacturer's instructions regarding any product used, but in this case the longer the solution is left in contact with the tooth, the deeper it will penetrate into the dentin. The goal of the dye is to assist you in locating the caries, not in determining how deep it goes. The depth will be determined by frequently checking dentin hardness with the explorer as you remove the softened dentin below the stain.

▪   Occasionally, after preparing a cavity and applying a caries disclosing dye, part of an internal (pulpal or axial) wall will stain. Carefully remove the stained dentin if you feel there is enough tooth structure below to prevent a pulp exposure. However, if you have doubts as to whether a pulp exposure may occur and the pulp is healthy (tooth asymptomatic), consider not removing the stained dentin. If you do, a pulp exposure may occur increasing the chances of the tooth becoming symptomatic and needing RCT. The stained dentin may or may not be infected. If it is infected, studies show that the placement of a well-sealed restoration can prevent the caries from progressing.[6] Place

---

5 Masatoshi Nakajima, Sitthikorn Kunawarote, Taweesak Prasansuttiporn, Junji Tagami. Bonding to caries affected dentin. *Japanese Dental Science Review*. 2011 Aug; 47(2):102–114

6 Thompson V, et al. Treatment of deep carious lesions by complete excavation or partial removal: A critical review. *J Am Dent Assoc*. 2008 Jun; 139(6): 705–712.

Dycal (Dentsply, York, PA) over the thin and stained areas of the internal walls, cover this with a glass ionomer (GI) liner in order to prevent dislodgement of the Dycal during the restorative procedure, and restore the tooth as you normally would. Warn the patient that the restoration went very close to the pulp and that eventually the tooth may need RCT.

▪ When using a caries disclosing dye, do not apply it in excess. Try to keep it only within the cavity preparation. This will prevent it from staining the restorations in adjacent teeth. Normally, caries disclosing dyes do not stain adjacent restorations but, on occasion, this can happen.[7]

Deciding Which Restorative Treatment to Use

After removing all caries and the areas of thin or undermined enamel, determine what are the restorative options for the tooth. The options normally are a direct composite, an inlay or onlay, or a crown.

❖ In the past, when amalgam was the restorative material of choice, the rule was that if a cusp was being replaced, the treatment options were either a metal onlay or a crown. The reason for this was that the unsupported amalgam could easily fracture. Currently, with the excellent quality of new resin composite materials, the treatment options for this type of situation are not as clear cut anymore. Longitudinal studies show that a direct composite restoration can successfully replace a missing cusp, and also that the prognosis for a cusp replacement restoration is similar for direct and indirect composites.[8] The onlay, whether it is made of resin composite, porcelain or metal, is costlier at present and more time consuming to the patient than a direct composite restoration. Therefore, it seems to me that, in

---

7 Harorli OT, et al. Caries detector dyes: Do they stain only the caries? Journal of Restorative Dentistry, 2014 Jan–Apr; 2(1): 20 - 26

8 Plotino G, et al. Fracture resistance of endodontically treated molars restored with extensive composite resin restorations. *J Prostheci Dent.* 2008 Mar; 99(3):225-32; Fennis W, Kuijs R, Roeters F, Creugers N, Kreulen C. Randomized Control Trial of Composite Cuspal Restorations: Five-year Results. *J Dent Res.* 2014 Jan; 93(1): 36–41

most cases where not much tooth structure is missing, a direct composite is a better option for cusp replacement than an onlay.

❖   When faced with a cusp replacement on a vital tooth, check how much tooth structure is left. If the restoration is shallow, although it involves a cusp, a direct composite is a good alternative.[9] On the other hand, a crown seems to have a better prognosis when, besides replacing a cusp, the restoration is deep, involves more than 50% of the coronal tooth structure and/or has subgingival interproximal boxes. When deciding which treatment to recommend, take into consideration the magnitude of the masticatory forces (big, well developed masticatory muscles versus small muscles) and any detrimental factors which may be present, such as, bruxism, a history of clenching and a history of fractured teeth and restorations. In border line cases, stronger muscles and presence of detrimental factors tip the scale towards the placement of a crown. The opposite tips the scale towards a direct restoration.

After deciding which treatment is the better option, explain to the patient its advantages and disadvantages compared with the alternative (a direct composite conserves tooth structure, costs less but is not as strong as a crown and, therefore, may not last as long), and why you recommend it over the other choice.

❖   A situation in which a gold onlay is an excellent restorative option is when a cusp needs to be replaced in a patient with strong masticatory muscles, a history of fractured teeth and restorations, and where the amount of tooth structure to be replaced is relatively small. The gold onlay is a strong restoration that when well made, can last for decades.[10] A direct resin composite replacing a cusp, in such a patient, would not have as favorable a prognosis. A gold crown, on the other hand, would

9 Deliperi S, Bardwell D. Clinical evaluation of direct cuspal coverage with posterior composite resin restorations. *J Esthet Restor Dent.* 2006; 18(5):256-65. Staehle H, et al. More conservative dentistry: clinical long-term results of direct composite resin restorations. *Quintessence Int.* 2015 May; 46(5):373-80.
10 Bandlish L, Mariatos G. Long-term survivals of 'direct-wax' cast gold onlays: a retrospective study in a general dental practice. *Br Dent J.* 2009 Aug 8; 207(3):111-5. Donovan T1, Simonsen RJ, Guertin G, Tucker RV. Retrospective clinical evaluation of 1,314 cast gold restorations in service from 1 to 52 years. *J Esthet Restor Dent.* 2004;16(3):194-204.

have an equal prognosis, however, the tooth reduction required for it would be much more invasive than that for an onlay.

❖ Until there is conclusive evidence that endodontically treated posterior teeth restored only with a resin composite restoration have an equal or better survival rate than those restored with a crown, it seems to me that it still is in the best interest of the patient to have such teeth restored with a crown.[11]

❖ Sometimes there is so little coronal tooth structure left after the removal of an old restoration, caries and unsupported enamel that, even though the tooth is vital, the indicated treatment is RCT, core build up and a crown. It can happen that the patient cannot afford this treatment at that moment. When this is the case, one may offer the patient the option of a direct composite. However, it is important to make it clear to him that the restoration is to be considered a good temporary. Explain that the tooth may become symptomatic and also that the restoration can fracture or come off at any moment (this is especially true in anterior teeth when there is extensive coronal destruction, and the bonded surface is small in comparison with the size of the restoration). Make a notation in the patient's records of what you told the patient and of what he said to you. When the patient is ready to have the RCT, core build up and crown done, consider not charging for the core build up, since the patient has already paid for the restoration.

❖ When, during an exam, one detects caries at a crown margin, the treatment of choice is always to remove the crown to clearly see the extent of the caries and then to fabricate a new crown. However, if the patient cannot afford a new crown at that moment, one may consider leaving the present crown in place and placing a restoration at the margin. A good candidate for this treatment option would be a patient with low caries activity and in which the caries at the crown margin appears to be small. The treatment consists in grinding, with a high-speed round diamond bur, the portion of the crown margin that is covering the caries in order to better see the cavity, removing the carious

11 Tikku AP, et al. Are full cast crowns mandatory after endodontic treatment in posterior teeth? *J Conserv Dent*. 2010 Oct-Dec; 13(4): 246–248.

lesion, and placing a restoration. One may consider amalgam as a restorative material because its corrosion products will have a sealing effect on the margins.[12] Before starting the treatment it is important to warn the patient that this is a "patch job" and that, whenever he can afford it, a new crown should be made.

❖   Occasionally, especially in the posterior areas, a patient will present with an edentulous space which, due to tooth movement, does not match the width of his teeth on the contralateral side. For example, the patient is missing tooth #30, yet the space between #29 and #31 is smaller than the width of #19. Or, sometimes, a molar and premolar are missing but the space left is not quite wide enough for a molar and premolar. In cases such as these, consider having the dental laboratory do a diagnostic wax up of the tooth (teeth) that is being replaced. The upper and lower models, along with the bite registration, are sent to the lab and the technician then waxes a tooth (teeth) in the edentulous area. The purpose of this is so that both you and the patient may visualize what the tooth replacement can look like and adjust it according to your wish before a definitive restoration is made.

A diagnostic wax up of missing teeth is especially useful in implant cases. It not only helps the patient visualize what the final restoration will look like, as he decides whether to undergo a costlier treatment, but also serves as a guide for the fabrication of a stent for the surgical placement of the implants.

❖   If you feel bleaching is indicated prior to performing a restorative treatment, explain to the patient about the types of bleaching, from over-the-counter products to in office bleaching. Explain that bleaching dispensed by the dentist costs more but obtains quicker results than over the counter products.

---

12 Ben-Amar A, et al. The sealing of the tooth/amalgam interface by corrosion products. J Oral Rehabil. 1995 Feb;22(2):101-4.

Prognosis

❖   Determining the prognosis of a restoration is a somewhat subjective effort. It depends on: the patient's eating habits; whether he has parafunctional habits (such as clenching); caries risk; the amount of tooth structure left and where in the tooth is located the greater bulk of this tooth structure, such as the buccal or lingual surface of an anterior tooth (a maxillary incisor with the greater bulk of tooth structure on the lingual has a better prognosis than if it is on the buccal due to the direction of the forces applied to the incisal edge in protrusive movements); the patient's chewing forces; periodontal condition; quality of oral hygiene; systemic conditions and medications which affect salivary flow, etc. One must take all this into consideration before arriving at a prognosis.

❖   Prior to starting any treatment, make sure the patient understands it, its prognosis, the pros and cons in comparison with other treatment options, and the cost. Make a note in the patient's chart that you have explained this to him.

❖   When giving a prognosis, always point out, within a realistic frame, the most negative scenario. For example, when discussing a treatment denture (flipper), explain: "This is a temporary treatment, and it may not last 6 months. It can break before then if you aren't careful with it". It is always better to realistically lower the patient's expectations and have a case exceed them than to have the opposite happen. Even if this means that some patients will decline a treatment due to its poor prognosis. By taking this approach, if there is a failure, the patient will understand because he has been forewarned. On the other hand, if the treatment does better than predicted, the patient will feel it was a good investment of his time and money.

❖   From my personal experience, a couple of factors that will make the prognosis guarded for a composite restoration: (1) very large restoration replacing more than 50% of coronal tooth structure, (2) large restoration replacing all the incisal edge.

❖   Some of the factors related to chewing forces that help determine the prognosis of a restoration on a tooth with extensive coronal destruction are: whether the patient has a history of restorations and teeth fracturing; the strength of patient's bite; the type of antagonist—if the tooth occludes against a complete denture or a distal extension RPD, the tendency is for less force to be applied to it than if it occludes against a natural tooth or an implant supported restoration.

❖   Occasionally, prior to preparing a tooth for a crown, a crown lengthening surgery will be necessary to prevent invasion of the biologic width. When this is the case, before starting the treatment, explain to the patient what is involved and the prognosis. Depending on the case the prognosis could range from good, such as in a single rooted premolar with a deep distal interproximal box, but with plenty of coronal tooth structure left, to guarded, such as in a molar with just enough tooth structure left for a ferrule around its circumference and in which the crown lengthening procedure will come close to exposing the furcation. When the prognosis is guarded, you can give the patient a time frame such as, "We can try to save this tooth, but the treatment may not last more than a couple of years because there is not much tooth structure left". In this case, factors which would improve the prognosis and tip the balance in favor of presenting the possibility of maintaining the tooth (though with a guarded prognosis) would be good resistance to periodontal disease (no history of periodontal disease—healthy bone level throughout the dental arches), excellent oral hygiene, low to absent caries activity, low bite forces, and a motivated patient. The reason for offering this option to the patient is that few people want to have a tooth extracted if there is hope of keeping it, even if for a limited period of time. Some may have insurance that covers a good portion of the treatment; others may be able to afford it despite the risk of losing the tooth within a couple of years. Write in the chart what you said to the patient and what he said to you.

Chapter 5

RESIN COMPOSITE RESTORATION

Materials & Instruments

The materials one uses when doing restorative treatment have a big part to play in the long term success of the restoration. One can have perfect tooth preparation and restoration placement techniques but, if the materials used are of poor quality, problems such as excessive wear, fractures, or tooth sensitivity may occur. It is very important, therefore, to choose good quality materials.

As a rule, the good quality materials are the more expensive ones. They are well worth the investment, however, since less time will be spent in fixing the problems that can arise from the use of low quality products, and one will have the personal satisfaction of having placed beautiful, lasting restorations.

A way to find out which materials to use is to ask your dental supplies salesperson what the dentists who have fee for service practices are using. Once you have this information, look up studies comparing the physical properties of these materials. The unbiased studies are usually those published in peer reviewed journals, where the authors have no commercial interest in the products researched. And, while we are in the topic of reading dental studies, please allow me to add an additional piece of advice: a good general rule when studying or reading anything related to science (including these notes) is to apply critical thinking. That is, a healthy dose of skepticism. Just because someone wrote it, does not mean it is correct. It can be correct or incorrect. Analyzing the materials and methods section of a study helps one to determine if its conclusions are valid.

Resin composites and bonding agents have been constantly changing over the last several years. Often a new and improved product is made available in the market. Therefore, it is a good idea to make it a point to keep oneself up to date on new developments in this area. Belonging to a study group is one way to keep abreast of changes.

❖   **Instrument Lubricating Agents**. When placing a restoration, it is important that the resin composite not stick to the placement instrument. If it sticks, it takes longer to place the material in the cavity, voids can be created, and the whole procedure can get a little frustrating. It can be like when one is trying to place a Band-Aid over a cut but it sticks to the wrong part of the finger. Several manufacturers claim to have non-stick instruments, but I have yet to find one that lives up to this claim.   However, there are lubricating agents available that work very well for this purpose. They are made specifically for wetting the placement instrument to prevent the composite from sticking to it and have no deleterious effect on the restorative material such as do alcohol or bonding agents which contain a solvent. A search phrase for this product is: "resin composite placement instrument lubricant. "

A way of using the lubricant: Place a drop on a container and, before placing the instrument on the composite, dip it into the lubricating agent. Remove any excess with a gauze sponge or by wiping the instrument on the patient's bib.

❖   **#12 scalpel blade.** Use it to finish the margins of every restoration that involves an interproximal surface. It removes excess material that may be present at the gingival cavosurface margin, leaving a smooth transition from tooth to restoration. It is important, however, not to grow overconfident in its use. If one's hand carelessly slips, the scalpel can cause great damage, cutting deeply the soft tissue. Use it calmly, slowly and with the ring finger and little finger firmly braced on the adjacent teeth. Floss after using the #12 scalpel blade. If the floss gets caught at the cervical area, it is usually a sign that there is still excess composite at the margin. When this happens, use the #12 scalpel blade again, followed by rechecking the area with floss.

❖   **332 carbide bur.** Great to remove amalgam. It cuts it like butter. Use a new one for each patient. Keeping a little box full of these at close reach of the assistant will save chair time. There is a difference in the cutting   efficiency   of   carbide   burs   fabricated   by   different manufacturers.[1] If you feel the bur you use does not cut very well, try another brand. Midwest (Dentsply, Switzerland) is an example of a good quality brand for this type of bur.

❖ **Round diamond burs.** Useful in removing caries and shaping the cavity. There are different diameters that fit well the different cavity sizes. A composite bur kit should include one bur each of sizes 2, 4 and 6. Round carbides work, but they tend to crack thin enamel when they are slightly dull. Diamonds are more expensive but remain sharp longer and only rarely will cause a crack on enamel.

❖ **Football shaped burnisher.** Useful in carving the occlusal anatomy.

❖ **Tofflemire matrix.** Works well for posterior teeth and canines. There are cases, such as when the interproximal cavity is small, where a sectional matrix band is easier and quicker to use.

❖ **Small flat instrument, such as Hu-Friedy 11 composite instrument** (Hu-Friedy Mfg. Co., Chicago, IL). Excellent for non-carious cervical lesions (NCCL) and for anterior composites

❖ **Large flat instrument.** Useful when placing a large Class IV restoration.

❖ **Serrated strip.** Used to separate the teeth if you are not able to floss the interproximal space after placing a composite restoration. The serrated strip will remove hardened composite, bonding agent, or cement which may inadvertently have overflowed into the interproximal space. It has smooth sides and has a cutting edge like a saw. It will not abrade or roughen the interproximal surfaces.

❖ **Sof-Lex Discs** (3M ESPE Dental, St Paul, MN). These are very good for finishing and polishing the buccal surfaces of anterior teeth.

---

1 Di Cristofaro R, Giner L, Mayoral J. Comparative Study of the Cutting Efficiency and Working Life of Carbide Burs. *Journal of Prosthodontics.* 2013, 22: 391–396. Note – This study was supported by Coltene/Whaledent, the manufacturer of one of the burs tested in this study. Another source is http://www.aapd.org/assets/1/25/Wilwerding-12-03.pdf.

Before Preparing the Cavity

❖   When placing a restoration, the first step is to select the shade. If the treatment has been started and the tooth is dry by the time it is selected, once the tooth moistens again its shade will change and there will be a poor color match between tooth and restoration.

❖   Administer profound anesthesia. On maxillary teeth, when an interproximal wedge must be used, numb the interdental papilla as well. This is a very sensitive area, but the injection can be painless if one waits for the infiltrative anesthesia administered earlier to have its effect. Once the tooth and buccal gingiva are numb one can, from the buccal, numb the interdental papilla without causing any pain.

❖   Check the occlusion prior to starting the treatment. This will give you an idea of what shape the occlusal surface of the restoration will have, saving finishing time. For example: if the opposing cusps are small and rounded, you will know your restoration does not need to have deep grooves and steep cusp inclinations.

Preparing the Cavity

❖   Be careful to grind with the bur only as deep as the caries goes. The closer the preparation is to the pulp, the greater the resulting pulpal inflammation.[2]

❖   **Ask the patient if he is feeling pain** while you drill or when you place an interproximal wedge. Watch his face and hands for signs of discomfort while you are working. If the patient grimaces ever so slightly, closes his eyes tightly, or clenches the armrests with his fingers, stop and ask, "Is it hurting?" If so, administer more anesthesia.

❖   When there is a pulp exposure and the pulp is healthy, obtain hemostasis, cover the exposure with Dycal (Dentsply, York, PA)

---

2 About I, Murray PE, Franquin JC, Remusat M, Smith AJ. Pulpal inflammatory responses following non-carious class V restorations. Oper Dent. 2001 Jul-Aug;26(4):336-42.

followed by a GI liner and place the definitive composite restoration. Advise the patient that there was a pulp exposure and enter in the chart a note that you have done so. In this case, as well as when there is no exposure but the restoration came very close to the pulp, or when the tooth restored presented initially with reversible pulpitis, warn the patient that the tooth may eventually need RCT, and explain in a few words what symptoms the patient should be on the lookout for. You can say, "It is normal if your tooth is a little sensitive to cold for the next few days. If it is sensitive, avoid whatever causes pain to give the nerve (pulp) a better chance to heal." You can explain that "An inflamed nerve is like a cut in the skin. Every time one drinks very cold liquids and causes the tooth to hurt it is as if one had a cut and scratched it. Just like scratching is an insult to the cut and will make it take longer to heal, drinking very cold liquids and causing the tooth to hurt is an insult to the nerve, but with a more severe consequence: the nerve may die and, as a result, the tooth will need a root canal."[3] Finally, warn the patient that, "If the tooth starts to hurt by itself, without your drinking cold liquids, it is a sign that the nerve is dying and you must come in for us to start the root canal." Years later, if the patient has pain, suspect this tooth.

❖ After caries removal on Class I and Class II cavities, do not leave overhanging occlusal enamel walls or very thin buccal, lingual, or interproximal walls. If left as they are, these thin walls and occlusal overhangs may fracture with time. It is better to remove a cusp than to leave a thin, undermined cusp.

❖ Consider placing a bevel on enamel when doing a Class IV composite restoration. This will improve retention and shade match.[4] The tapering form of the bevel provides a gradual shade and texture transition from the tooth to the composite.

---

3 Abd-Elmeguid A, Yu DC. Dental pulp neurophysiology: part 1. Clinical and diagnostic implications. *J Can Dent Assoc.* 2009 Feb; 75 (1):55-9.
4 Coelho-de-Souza F, et al. Influence of adhesive system and bevel preparation on fracture strength of teeth restored with composite resin. *Braz Dent J.* 2010;21(4):327-31. Coelho-de-Souza F, et al. Influence of restorative technique, beveling, and aging on composite bonding to sectioned incisal edges. *J Adhes Dent.* 2008 Feb;10(2):113-7.

❖   Always access the interproximal caries on an anterior tooth from the lingual surface to preserve a buccal enamel wall. This wall, even if only a thin shell, greatly improves the aesthetics of the restoration. The support given to the buccal enamel by the underlying resin composite is sufficient to protect it from fracturing. Usually there is no need for bevel placement on Class III restorations since the shape of the prepared cavity already contains an internal bevel.

❖   It is unnecessary to place a bevel when restoring a non-carious cervical lesion since its shape is a bevel in itself.

Resin Composite Placement

❖   Always use a wedge when it is an interproximal restoration. Place it so that it is tight. This will accomplish two things besides preventing overflow of composite into the interproximal space: (1) It will help to prevent bleeding and therefore assist in keeping the cavity dry. (2) In teeth with normal mobility (1 or less), it will cause a slight separation between them which, in turn, will lead to a tighter contact once the wedge is removed and the teeth rebound to their original position. It usually takes a few minutes for the teeth to shift back and for the contact to tighten.

❖   In teeth with more than 1 mobility, one must be careful when placing the interproximal wedge. If one pushes the wedge in too tightly, the pressure may cause a separation between the teeth greater than the minimal separation desired. The restoration will fill the created space, will be wider than it should be and will prevent the teeth from shifting back to their original position. This change in tooth position will likely interfere with the occlusion and it can be unaesthetic. When the tooth being restored has more than 1 mobility, place the wedge very carefully, without using much pressure and watching to see if there is excessive lateral tooth movement.

❖   A way of obtaining a nice, tight interproximal contact and good composite adaptation to the interproximal walls: Fill the interproximal box with composite, insert the condenser (after dipping it into the lubricating agent and wiping the excess off) into the composite pushing it in a cervical direction, then 1 or 2 mm in a buccal direction followed by 1or 2 mm in a lingual direction. Excess material will flow over the occlusal margin. Remove the excess with your condenser and wipe the instrument with a gauze sponge. Place the condenser again into the composite (lubricate if you feel it is necessary), push 1 or 2 mm cervically and then push the instrument against the matrix in a horizontal (mesial or distal) direction. Cure the composite with the condenser in this position. Apply the light for an extra 20 seconds or so in order to partially cure the composite immediately below the instrument. Remove the condenser and cure the composite again in order to finish polymerizing the area that was covered by the instrument during the initial cure. After this initial fill, the matrix will be tightly held against the adjacent tooth by the cured composite. One can then proceed to fill the remaining interproximal and occlusal areas in the conventional manner.

The necessary shape for a condenser, in this case, is that its nib (working end) be slightly conical, with the narrower end at the face (tip) of the instrument. This shape will prevent it from getting trapped when you cure the initial layer of composite at the interproximal box with the condenser in the composite. This shape also assists in pushing the composite against the buccal and lingual interproximal walls.

❖ When the cavity preparation ends close to the pulp, protect the pulp with Dycal (Dentsply, York, PA). There is no need to cover the entire internal wall, just the area close to the pulp, so as to leave more dentin exposed and available for bonding. Cover the Dycal (Dentsply, York, PA) with a light cured GI cement to protect it from dislodgement caused by the etching, rinsing, and bonding agent application procedures.

❖ The resin composite can occasionally start curing (hardening) before one is finished placing it, depending on the brand of resin composite one is using, the intensity of the dental chair light, and the length of time one is taking to pack the material into the cavity. A way to prevent this from happening is to have a dental chair light with variable light intensity and to set it at its lowest intensity just prior to inserting the resin composite. If the dental chair light you use has only one light intensity, another option for preventing this problem from occurring is to turn the beam of light away from the tooth just as you start inserting the material. If one is using magnification, one can still see well enough with ambient light to finish condensing the resin composite into the preparation even though the chair light is not illuminating it directly. The dental assistant can be trained to dim the light or turn it away at the appropriate time.

Adjusting the Occlusion

After placing a restoration, take your time adjusting the occlusion. It is important that the restoration not be high. A high restoration can become uncomfortable to the patient once the anesthesia wears off and may eventually cause reversible pulpitis along with sensitivity to chewing.[5] The patient has then to return to your office for further adjustment. Both you and he end up spending additional time on this tooth. As far as problems go, a high restoration is not the most serious and it can happen with any dentist, but it is better if it can be avoided. Also, in the patient's mind, it can be seen as a mistake on the dentist's part.

❖   Some patients will not tell you that the restoration feels high unless you ask, "Does it feel high?" If you ask, "Does it feel okay?" a few patients will answer, "Yes," because they don't want to be thought of as a complainer and/or because they believe the weird feeling they have when they bite down (the high restoration) is caused by the anesthesia and will go away with time. Always make the question specific such as "Does it feel high?" or, "When you close, does it feel that the tooth we worked on is hitting first—before the others touch?"

❖   Before adjusting the occlusion, look again at the occlusal anatomy of the opposing tooth. This will remind you of what the anatomy of the

5 Clark G, Tsukiyama Y, Baba K, Watanabe T. Sixty-eight years of experimental occlusal interference studies: what have we learned? *J Prosthet Dent.* 1999 Dec; 82(6):704-13.

restoration you just placed should look like, and will speed up the adjustment process.

❖   Adjust the occlusion in small increments, using a football shaped diamond bur. Excessive grinding may leave a large space between the occlusal surfaces of opposing teeth, where sticky food can accumulate when the patient eats. The reason for the diamond bur is that, in my experience, carbide burs (other than multifluted finishing burs), when dull, tend to produce cracks in the restoration or tooth structure. The reason for the football shape is that it creates a more aesthetic, smoother anatomy than a round bur.

❖   Do not rely solely on the patient's input when you are adjusting the occlusion. His judgement is impaired by the anesthesia. Ask him if the restoration feels high only after you don't see any more premature contacts when checking with the articulating paper. If he states it is high, check with the articulating paper again. Ask him to, "Bite a little harder and grind your teeth a little." Usually, one will find an area that was high and had not yet been adjusted.

❖   If you check the occlusion, adjust once, and before checking again ask the patient if it is high, it will likely still be high and (hopefully) he will answer, "Yes." After repeating this process about 4 or 5 times, with the patient having to answer as many times that it is still high, both you and the patient will start to feel uncomfortable with each other. Eventually, he may say it is fine just to put an end to the awkward situation even though the restoration may still feel high. The same patient will not mind, however, if you do not say anything besides, "Open please," and, "Bite down please," while checking the occlusion, adjusting the restoration, checking the occlusion again, adjusting again, and repeating this a few times until you see there are no more premature contacts and, only then, ask him if it feels high.

❖   Sometimes, when applying a jet of air to a prepared cavity as part of the bonding procedure, a drop of bonding agent will spill onto the occlusal surface of a neighboring tooth. This drop, if thick enough, may create a premature contact and will be marked by the articulating paper. If there are no contacts on the restoration you just placed, and the patient still feels that it is high, the spilled bonding agent may be the cause. Run a dull, multifluted finishing bur over the areas marked with the articulating paper on the adjacent teeth. If there is any bonding agent that is interfering with occlusion, this should remove it without reducing the tooth structure.

❖   Have the patient do protrusive movements when you are adjusting the occlusion after placing a Class IV restoration. Make sure there is no interference in this movement, or the restoration may come off within a short period of time.

❖   Use 5 mm width strips of articulating paper when you don't want an occlusal contact in a certain area of the tooth. This allows you to check the occlusion section by section. If the teeth do not grip the articulating paper, it is because there is no contact in that area.

Finishing and Polishing

❖   The better polished the restoration is, the less plaque adhesion.[6]

❖   A simple way to finish and polish composites done on posterior teeth and the lingual surfaces of anterior teeth is with a dull, multifluted finishing bur followed by a rubber polishing tip. The reason to use a dull bur is because it will not alter the shape of the restoration.

❖   In a posterior tooth, even if it is just an occlusal restoration, run a dull, multifluted finishing bur over its buccal and lingual surfaces as part of the finishing and polishing process. This is done in order to remove any excess, sharp composite or adhesive which inadvertently may have spilled there, and which may bother the patient once the anesthesia wears off. It will only take about 5 seconds to do this and it may save the patient some discomfort later on and a resultant additional visit to take care of the problem.

❖   Always floss after finishing a restoration. This will allow you to determine whether: (1) the contact is adequate; (2) there are overhangs at the margins of the restoration. If the floss catches at the cervical

---

6 Vyavahare N, et al. Effect of finishing and polishing procedures on biofilm adhesion to composite surfaces: An ex vivo study. *J Dent Allied Sci* 2014;3:70-3

margins of the restoration, it is a sign that there are overhangs. When this happens, use the #12 scalpel blade again to remove the excess composite at the interproximal margin. After removing the excess material, floss one more time to make sure the restoration is adequate.

❖ Even if the restoration does not extend into the interproximal surface, flossing should be a part of the finishing routine. It will either remove any excess composite or adhesive which may inadvertently have filled that area or, if the floss does not go through, it will show you there is a blocked contact. In the latter case, a serrated strip will remove the excess material allowing the floss to pass the contact.

❖ Sometimes, immediately after placing a Class II composite restoration, you may feel that the contact is light when you check it with the floss. Do not redo the interproximal box straightaway. Wait a few minutes or check again at the next visit. The interproximal wedge slightly separates the tooth being restored from the adjacent tooth. The light contact may be the result of the teeth not yet having completely rebounded to their original position. If this is the case, with time, as the teeth shift back, the contact will tighten.

❖ If there is no interproximal contact at all between neighboring posterior teeth after you place a Class II restoration, then it is best to prepare a proximal box into the just placed restoration and redo the contact area before dismissing the patient. The same applies to anterior teeth unless aesthetics requires that you leave a space, such as when the patient has diastemas and wants to keep it that way.

❖ After placing a Class IV composite restoration make sure you remove all material that goes beyond the beveled margin. If one is not careful, a thin veneer of composite can remain at this area and extend a few millimeters over the buccal surface. If there has been no bonding between this veneer and the tooth structure, with time an unaesthetic stain may form below it. At other times, the veneer may chip off leaving an uncomfortable step in the restoration.

Post Op Instructions

❖   After placing a large restoration, warn the patient he may feel pain to chewing and to cold. If the restoration is close to the pulp, warn him that the tooth treated may eventually need RCT due to the proximity of the restoration to the pulp. Explain to the patient the symptoms of irreversible pulpitis so that he may know what to look for. Your explanation can be clear and simple, such as, "The filling went very close to the nerve and there is a chance the tooth may end up needing a root canal. If the tooth starts to hurt by itself, or if it takes too long for the pain to subside after you drink cold water, it is a sign that the nerve is dying. If this happens, you need to come in so that we can take care of the pain and start the root canal." Make an entry in your chart of what you told the patient. Also, tell the patient to avoid whatever causes pain on the treated tooth. "If it hurts with cold, avoid cold".

Restoring Non-Carious Cervical Lesions (NCCLs)

❖   Insert a retraction cord moistened with a hemostatic solution in the gingival sulcus. Place it along the entire buccal surface extending a couple of millimeters into the mesial and distal surfaces. This will help prevent bleeding from the surrounding gingiva while you carve the restoration.

❖   Take your time and carve the restoration well, with a small flat instrument such as the Hu-Friedy 11 composite instrument, in order to prevent excess material from extending beyond the cervical margin. The coronal margin of the restoration is not as critical since it is simpler to finish, being far from the gingiva. After curing the composite, run the explorer over the margins of the restoration in order to determine if there are any overhangs. If there is any excess composite along the cervical margins of the restoration, avoid removing it with a bur because the bur can nick the tooth and/or gingiva. The excess material can be removed with small diameter Sof-Lex (3M ESPE Dental, St Paul, MN) discs or a #12 scalpel blade. When using the Sof-Lex discs, protect the gingiva with the large flat instrument (from the composite kit). The disc does not damage the instrument. Removing excess from the coronal margin of the restoration can also be done with the discs.

❖   In general, good shades for cervical composite restorations are Filtek Supreme A (1, 2 or 3, depending on the shade of the tooth) B (3M ESPE Dental, St Paul, MN).

❖   Do not leave a retraction cord in the gingival sulcus for more than 10 minutes, as this may burn the gingiva causing discomfort to the patient and possible recession.[7]

❖   Warn the patient that the gingiva may be sore due to the use of the retraction cord and recommend rinse with warm water and salt 2 or 3 times a day for a couple of days if it is sore.

---

7 Liu CM, Huang FM, Yang LC, Chou LS, Chou MY, Chang YC. Cytotoxic effects of gingival retraction cords on human gingival fibroblasts in vitro. *J Oral Rehabil*. 2004 Apr;31(4):368-72.

Chapter 6

CROWN

Before Starting

❖ Prior to starting a crown preparation remember always to check the occlusion. By checking the occlusion, you will have an idea of how much tooth structure needs to be removed, and where on the tooth it needs to be removed, to obtain adequate space for the crown material being used, such as 1.5 mm occlusal space for a PFM crown or 2 mm incisal space for an all-porcelain crown. This is especially useful in posterior teeth when the tooth being treated has a short clinical crown that may not provide much retention and resistance if further reduced.

Often, in a posterior tooth, not all occlusal areas need to be reduced by the same amount to obtain an even clearance, 1.5 mm for example. This is because the shape of the opposing tooth/teeth does not always mesh perfectly with the occlusal surface being prepared. A way to check how much tooth reduction is needed in each area of the occlusal surface is, prior to starting the procedure, to have the patient bite on a strip of wax. The imprint left by the teeth on the wax will allow you to see exactly where, and how much, tooth reduction is needed to obtain an even clearance.

❖ If a tooth needing a crown has advanced bone loss, even if there is no active periodontal disease, consider referring the patient to a periodontist to determine the prognosis and whether a crown may be placed.

❖ While choosing the shade for a crown on an incisor, pay attention to the incisal edges of its neighboring incisors. Often, especially in older persons, the incisal edges are very translucent. Not bluish, as some lab technicians would like to make it, but transparent. If you put an instrument or your gloved finger on the lingual side of the incisor, you can see it from the buccal side. Make a note of the length of the translucent section in an incisal apical direction, usually it is between 1 and 2 mm, and write it on the lab prescription. You can also make a drawing of the buccal surface and trace on it the transparent section at the incisal edge. Let the technician know that you want that area transparent. When it is a quality lab, the resulting porcelain crown will look very natural and will beautifully match the neighboring teeth.

❖ Before preparing a crown, remember to have quality, recent X-rays and to check the image for apical lesions and periodontal disease. This is obvious, but in the hustle and bustle of a busy day it can be overlooked.

❖ Place a crown on a tooth that has undergone periodontal surgery only after giving enough time for the gingival margins to stabilize. If the surgery included bone recontouring, one should wait a minimum of 3 months for posterior teeth before making the definitive crown preparation and as much as 6 months for teeth in the aesthetic zone.[1] Also in the aesthetic zone, if the surgery was minor and involved only gingiva, one should wait about 3 months.[2] If one does not wait for the gingiva to stabilize, one may place the margins subgingivally only for them to be exposed if the gingiva shrinks further.

❖ On an active patient, placement of a crown comes after all carious lesions and periodontal disease, if present, have been treated. Occasionally, however, a person who is not an active patient may come in needing a crown. An example of this would be someone who is residing temporarily in your city, or someone who was referred to you by another patient specifically for crown treatment. When this is the case, before starting the crown, remember always to do a general checkup for caries and periodontal disease as well to check the vitality of the tooth being treated. When there is caries and/or periodontal disease, these issues must be addressed along with the crown placement.

1 Hempton T, Dominici J. Contemporary crown-lengthening therapy: a review. *J Am Dent Assoc*. 2010 Jun; 141(6):647-55.
2 Afshar-Mohajer K, Stahl SS. The remodeling of human gingival tissues following gingivectomy. *J Periodontol*. 1977 Mar; 48(3):136-9.

Which Materials to Use

❖   When deciding which materials to use for crown cementation, impressions, bite registration, temporary crown fabrication, etc., a good starting point is to ask your dental supply salesperson which ones are popular with the fee for service practices. Then, armed with this information, look up peer reviewed studies on the recommended materials. Studies in journals such as *JADA*, *Quintessence International*, *General Dentistry* (published by the Academy of General Dentistry), where the authors have no commercial interest in the materials being researched.

❖   If the patient has a strong bite, tends to break teeth and restorations, and the tooth needing a crown is a molar, consider placing a gold crown. This applies especially to someone who is not overly concerned about aesthetics. The gold crown will not fracture, has great margins, and does not produce excessive wear on the opposing dentition. Also, it requires less tooth reduction than a porcelain fused to metal crown (PFM).

❖   Consider using a yellow colored alloy (with a high content of gold) for PFM crowns. Crowns will then be much more aesthetic, especially along the cervical area where porcelain is thinner, since gold mimics dentin better than the silver colored alloys.

❖   For maxillary incisors, in most cases, the treatment of choice is an all-porcelain crown. Systems that utilize feldspathic glass porcelain are usually very aesthetic and have adequate strength if bonded to the tooth structure as opposed to cementing the crown with glass ionomer cement.[3]

❖   For lower incisors, consider a PFM crown, since it requires less tooth reduction than an all-porcelain crown, allowing for a thicker, stronger tooth core.

❖   Choose a set of specific burs that you like and stick to them. The reason to continue with the same size and type of burs is that by using

---

3 Kelly JR.Dental ceramics: current thinking and trends. *Dent Clin North Am*. 2004 Apr; 48(2):viii, 513-30.

the same burs, in the same manner, repeatedly, you will develop a crown preparation routine. Having this routine will greatly speed up the restorative process.

A wide, extra course, tapered round end diamond bur (for example: bur #856-025) is well suited for the buccal, lingual, and occlusal surfaces because it reduces tooth structure more quickly than a thinner bur. When it is time to reduce the interproximal surfaces and, if necessary, place the margins subgingivally, a thin, extra course, tapered round end bur (for example: bur #856-014) is indicated because it will prevent damage to the neighboring teeth and gingiva. When the type of crown being placed requires a shoulder margin, one may use an extra course, tapered flat end bur (for example: bur #847-018). A fine grit bur of each respective size can be used to smooth the walls of the preparation after tooth reduction is completed.[4] Multifluted carbide burs may also be used for finishing. A smoothly finished preparation will facilitate lab work and provide a better fitting crown.

❖   There are sets of finishing and polishing rubber tips made specifically for porcelain which one can use after doing adjustments on a porcelain fused to metal (PFM) crown or an all-porcelain crown.

Communicating with the Patient

❖   As you explain crown treatment to the patient, show him finished cases of the different types of crowns (PFM with metal collar on lingual, metal collar all around, porcelain covered margins all around; all porcelain crown, gold crown) that you have waiting to be delivered or that you have specifically for patient instruction. This will help him visualize and understand your explanation.

❖   If you see that the patient is overly concerned with aesthetics, when explaining about crown treatment for a maxillary incisor it is prudent to warn the patient that, "The shade and translucency will not be exactly equal to that of the adjacent natural incisor. It will be similar but not

---

4 http://www.ffofr.org/education/lectures/fixed-prosthodontics/fixed-prosthodontics-tooth-preparation-guidelines-for-complete-coverage-metal-crowns

exactly equal." When you tell him this, you are realistically lowering the patient's expectations. He will likely be more at peace with the results than he would have been if you had raised his expectations. If your warning leads him to decide to have the crown done somewhere else, perhaps it may be one less headache you will have.

❖ When doing a crown preparation on a vital tooth, always warn the patient that there is a possibility that the tooth may become sensitive to cold for a period of time. Also let him know that, even though it rarely occurs, this sensitivity may not improve with time, instead it may worsen, in which case the tooth will need RCT.[5]

❖ When you conclude that a crown will have a guarded prognosis, warn the patient that if he is not careful with what he eats or how he uses his teeth (such as using them to rip a plastic bag open), the crown may not last more than a couple of years. Let the patient decide if he wants to have the crown done. The other treatment option being extraction and replacement with an implant or another type of prosthesis.

❖ <u>While you are working, ask the patient if he feels pain</u>. If he says yes, stop and administer more anesthesia.

❖ Advise the patient that some mild discomfort following crown preparation is normal. Give the patient a small bottle of a chlorhexidine gluconate mouth rinse and recommend that he rinse for four days, starting the day the crown preparation is done. This will help to keep the gingiva healthy during the immediate post-operative period, when it may be painful to brush the area, and it will help to prevent a bleeding, irritated gingiva at the time of final cementation. The downside of this is that, occasionally, this type of rinse can stain the temporary crown and reversibly stain the teeth (a cleaning will remove the stains). As an alternative to rinsing with a chlorhexidine gluconate mouth rinse the patient may be instructed to rinse with warm water and salt, twice a day, for four days.

---

5 Hargraves K, Cohen S. Cohen's *Pathways of the Pulp*. Tenth Edition. Elsevier Publishing; 2011. Pp 516

Tooth Preparation

❖ When the opposing tooth has sharp centric cusps, consider rounding them slightly prior to taking the impression of the opposing arch. By rounding the opposing centric cusp slightly, the crown being made will not need to have very steep inclines and deep grooves. Steep inclines contribute to an increase in dislodging forces on the crown. The goal is for this crown to last a very, very long time and not to come off, ever.

❖ When the tooth that will be prepared for a crown is a posterior tooth with a short clinical crown and the opposing tooth is extruded, consider also reducing the occlusal surface of the opposing tooth. This will provide some of the space needed for the crown and allow for a longer, more retentive crown preparation. One must be careful, however, not to grind the opposing tooth excessively and expose dentin.

❖ Make sure the tooth being treated is completely numb before starting the crown preparation. Anesthetize both lingual and buccal gingiva well so that the patient does not feel pain when you place the retraction cord.

❖ Consider making it a habit of using a set of burs for a limited number of crown preparations (three to five). A sharp bur will save much time during tooth reduction and its cost is minimal if compared to the cost to the crown. The economy in time and reduced discomfort to the patient makes it well worth the small additional investment.

The finishing-polishing bur may be used several times since, when it is dull, it does not change the shape you have given to the preparation. It merely polishes it.

❖ In order to reduce as much as possible heat damage to the pulp, use abundant water spray while preparing a vital tooth. Sharp burs also reduce heat generation during crown preparation. These steps will help reduce post-operative pulpal inflammation and patient discomfort.[6]

---

6 Kwon S, et al. Thermal irritation of teeth during dental treatment procedures. *Restor Dent Endod.* 2013 Aug; 38(3):105-12.

❖   When you are working on a posterior tooth and there is not much clearance, use short shank burs so that the patient is not forced to open very wide. It can become uncomfortable to the patient if he has to spend several minutes with his mandible in a strained position.

❖   Always try to have direct vision of the surface you are preparing. Below are operator positions, given assuming the reader is right-handed. If left-handed, positions are opposite.

1) Interproximal surface of upper left posterior teeth: Go to the left side of the patient's chair. Have the patient face right side and close his mouth as much as possible while allowing clearance for the handpiece and bur. Place the patient chair low and in almost a horizontal position. This will normally give you direct vision when you retract the lip and approach from the buccal surface.

2) Lingual surface of upper right posterior teeth: Same position as above but with the difference that the patient must open wide.

3) Lower left posterior teeth: One may be able to see all surfaces from a position right behind the patient's head, that is, the 12 o'clock position.

4) Lower right posterior teeth: Same as lower left but also, for the mesial, distal, buccal, and occlusal surfaces you may prepare the tooth from a 9 o'clock position.

5) Lingual surface of maxillary anterior teeth: Have the patient lean his head to the left side and up. Place patient almost horizontally and stay at the 9 o'clock position.

6) Sometimes you can only see the distal of maxillary molars with the use of a mirror (using indirect vision). In these cases, have the patient open as wide as he can so that there is room for you to place the mirror in an area where the handpiece will not block the reflection of the interproximal surface. You may have the assistant spray air in your mirror to remove water droplets and provide better visibility while you prepare the tooth.

❖   It is only when there is absolutely no alternative that you should prepare a surface without being able to see the bur grinding the tooth. This can occur with the distal surface of the maxillary second molars in a person with a small mouth, where the mouth mirror (used for indirect vision) and the high-speed handpiece do not fit simultaneously. Prepare this surface last, after having reduced all other surfaces and having ground the distal buccal and distal lingual line angles as far as you can see. Usually only a 3 or 4 mm flat surface will be left for preparation, going from one prepared distal line angle to the other. As you prepare this area, stop frequently and look at the surface being ground to make sure it is assuming the shape you want.

❖   The internal angles of the crown preparation should be rounded and smooth. Rounded angles will facilitate lab work and reduce stress concentration on the definitive crown and on the temporary also.

❖   On maxillary incisors reduce the buccal surface in 2 planes following the natural curvature of the tooth. This will provide for better aesthetics.

❖   Make sure that the crown preparation has adequate resistance and retention forms. This is true especially for posterior teeth which can be wide and short. The long and thin shape of the coronal portion of anterior teeth lends itself to a retentive preparation. If the preparation does not have adequate retention and resistance forms, in one or two years the crown may come off. If necessary, extend the crown preparation as far subgingivally as healthy and/or, in posterior teeth, grind the opposing tooth (if the occlusal plane permits and if there will be no dentin exposure) in order to keep the preparation from being too short. Another option to increase resistance form in molars is to prepare a slot in the interproximal surfaces.

Retention form: is the ability of the preparation to resist the crown restoration from removal along its path of insertion.

Resistance form: is the ability of the preparation to resist the dislodgement of the restoration by forces directed obliquely or horizontally to the restoration.

❖   Do not invade biologic width. If this occurs: (1) the patient may have a constant chronic pain in the area or, more commonly, a discomfort/pain whenever the patient flosses or brushes; (2) there may be unpredictable bone loss in the area.[7]

❖   After tooth reduction, place the retraction cord in the sulcus and leave it for a couple of minutes. Then prepare the margins the way you want them. Use a bur that will not touch the gingiva. Usually, a thinner bur is indicated for this step. If the gingiva is touched with the bur: (1) The patient will have more postoperative discomfort; (2) it may be difficult to obtain an adequate final impression due to bleeding; (3) depending on the amount of damage to the soft tissue, there may be some recession.

Crown Margins

❖   Regardless of how well a crown margin fits the prepared tooth structure, there will be at least a microscopic ledge that will serve as a niche for the accumulation of bacteria. If resistance and retention forms, and aesthetics, do not require subgingival margins, consider placing the margins at gingival level or ever so slightly (0.3 mm) above it. Supragingival margins are more easily kept clean than subgingival margins, resulting in healthier gingiva and tooth structure.

❖   Regarding PFM crowns, in my experience, metal margins are usually flusher with the tooth structure than are porcelain covered margins or porcelain shoulders. When making a PFM crown, consider leaving a metal collar at areas that are not visible such as the lingual and distal margins. And if it is a tooth, such as a maxillary 2nd molar, where the margins will usually not be visible, no matter how hard the patient smiles, consider a metal collar all around the circumference of the crown. In this case, if you plan to have the margins in metal, it is prudent to advise the patient prior to preparing the tooth and explain the reason for your recommendation. Most patients understand and approve of the procedure. If a patient does not seem happy with the prospect of metal margins, the crown can have porcelain covered margins instead.

---

7 Newman G, Takei H. *Carranza's Clinical Periodontology.* Tenth Edition. Elsevier Pub; 2006. Pp. 1051 – 1052.

❖ The treatment of choice for a maxillary anterior tooth is usually an all-porcelain crown. However, when the amount of tooth reduction needed for an all-porcelain crown will leave a thin, weak core of tooth structure, a PFM crown may be a better option. When this is the case, consider a porcelain butt joint on the buccal surface. A quality lab will go a long way in making this type of crown have adequate margins. The use of a yellow gold alloy for the coping, in addition to the porcelain butt joint, and a quality lab, can result in a very aesthetic PFM crown.

Tissue Retraction

❖ Two common ways of retraction cord use:

1) Insert one retraction cord into the gingival sulcus, leave it in place for a few minutes and then remove it prior to taking the impression.

2) Insert two retraction cords into the gingival sulcus, a smaller diameter followed by a larger diameter cord. Remove the larger diameter cord and take the impression with the thinner cord still in the sulcus.

❖ With either technique, after removing the cord(s) spray water into the gingival sulcus in order to rinse away the chemicals present in the retraction cord.

❖ Soak the retraction cord in water before removing it from the sulcus. Pulling it while dry may tear the inner epithelial lining of the sulcus causing unwanted bleeding and trauma to the gingiva.

❖ When using the "one cord technique", after removing the cord and doing the impression, look for pieces of impression material in the sulcus.

❖ Do not leave the retraction cord in the gingival sulcus for longer than 10 minutes since, due to the chemicals used, this may burn the gingiva causing postoperative pain and, possibly, recession.[8]

---

8 Liu CM, Huang FM, Yang LC, Chou LS, Chou MY, Chang YC. Cytotoxic effects of gingival retraction cords on human gingival fibroblasts in vitro. *J Oral Rehabil.* 2004 Apr;31(4):368-72.

❖   Make a notation in the chart that you have placed and removed the retraction cord(s).

Impression – Bite Registration

❖   Inspect the impression closely. Make sure it shows all margins clearly, has no bubbles and depicts adjacent teeth and soft tissue well. If you are not sure the impression is adequate, it is best to retake it. The additional 5 to 10 minutes spent on this are little compared to the time and cost of having to fabricate a new crown because of inadequate margins that resulted from an inadequate impression. The least problem that can come from sending an inadequate impression to the dental laboratory is that the laboratory technician may call you and ask you to take a new impression, in which case it will have been time lost for you and time lost, discomfort and disappointment for the patient who must come back for an additional impression instead of for a crown delivery.

❖   Instead of using a triple tray and taking the final impression, opposing arch impression and bite registration all at the same time, consider obtaining these in separate steps. Start with an alginate impression of the opposing arch while waiting for the anesthesia to take effect, and take the bite registration after the crown prep, while the assistant polishes the temporary crown. The problem with the triple tray is that it has the potential of generating a distorted impression and an inaccurate bite registration. The tray itself may bend when the patient bites and rebound to its original position when he releases the pressure. Also, the mesh that separates upper and lower arches may interfere with the bite unless the patient manages to bite through it.[9]

❖   When taking the bite registration, place the patient's chair in an upright position. After covering the prepared tooth and adjacent teeth with bite registration material one can say to the patient: "Bite down with your back teeth, as if you were chewing a piece of steak."

---

9 http://www.dentalabstracts.com/article/S0011-8486(06)80393-6/fulltext

With an adequate bite registration, the lab can better articulate the models and, therefore, make a crown with an occlusal surface which will need less adjustment.

❖   The bite registration may capture the teeth in maximum intercuspation (MIP) if the patient does not suffer from temporomandibular joint disorder.[10] If the patient suffers from TMD, consider referring him to a dentist trained in its treatment prior to starting the crown.

❖   While taking the bite registration, sometimes the patient is tense, wants to help, and ends up biting edge to edge or in a position that you see is not MIP. If he is tense and having difficulty biting in MIP, tell him to close his mouth, swallow and bite as his teeth come close together. Explain that this is the position you want him to repeat when you place the bite registration material between his teeth.

❖   Check the case before sending it to the lab. Teach the assistants to pour the opposing model well, without bubbles and soon after the alginate impression is taken in order to avoid alginate distortion.

Temporary Crown

❖   Teach the assistant how to make a temporary crown. The temporary must: (1) have well adapted margins; (2) not interfere with occlusion; (3) have adequate interproximal contacts so as to prevent food impaction and an irritated, bleeding gingiva during definitive crown cementation; (4) and be well polished to reduce plaque adhesion and to be more comfortable to the patient. If the acrylic is rough, it can irritate the mucosa and the tongue.

❖   Consider using a non-eugenol temporary cement, such as TempBond NE (Kerr, Orange, CA), for the temporary crown. Eugenol has been shown to interfere with the bonding of resin composite to

---

10 Lila-Krasniqi ZD, et al. Differences between centric relation and maximum intercuspation as possible cause for development of temporomandibular disorder analyzed with T-scan III. *Eur J Dent.* 2015 Oct-Dec;9(4):573-9

tooth structure.[11] If a cement containing eugenol is used for the temporary crown, eugenol left on the tooth at the time of the definitive crown delivery may interfere with the bonding of a definitive resin cement to tooth structure.

❖   Advise the patient to floss at the temporary by pushing the floss through the contact, letting go one end and pulling the other end away from the mouth. This way the floss will go through the contact only in the direction of the gingiva, making it less likely to pull the crown away from the tooth. Explain that you used temporary cement and he must, therefore, be careful not to chew sticky foods or gum, otherwise the crown may come off.

❖   Advise the patient to call your office immediately if the temporary crown comes off. Warn him that if the temporary crown stays off for more than a day you may end up having to make a new crown. Without the temporary in place, the teeth may shift, and it may become difficult or impossible to fit the definitive crown.

❖   When the patient calls to let you know that the crown has come off, teach the employees what to tell him over the phone: 1) Ask the patient to come to the office at his earliest convenience, but on the same day, to recement the temporary. 2) Ask if the crown is intact, if so tell him to place it on the tooth, but to remove it prior to eating or drinking and to replace it afterwards.

❖   If the patient is working and can only come in after hours, consider staying late in order to recement a temporary crown that has come off.

The Dental Laboratory

❖   Use an excellent laboratory technician, even if his/her fees are high. A good laboratory technician will bring you much peace of mind as you go about your daily work. You will save time at the crown delivery appointment because his/her crowns will, in most cases: (1) have

11 Al Wazzan K, Al Harbi A, Hammad I. The Effect of Eugenol-Containing Temporary Cement on the Bond Strength of Two Resin Composite Core Materials to Dentin. *Journal of Prosthodontics.* 1997 March (6) 1: 37–42

interproximal contacts and occlusion that need very little adjustment; (2) be very aesthetic and pleasing to both patient and dentist; (3) have margins very faithful to what was captured in the impression.

❖ When one tries to save money in lab fees and uses a low quality lab, the crown delivery appointment can become an occasion that the dentist will come to dread with a passion. A lot of time may be spent on adjusting the interproximal contacts to get the crown to sit properly. Then, commonly there will be open margins, untrue to what was captured in the impression. If the margins turn out to be acceptable, when the patient and dentist check the aesthetics, they may often find the crown just plain ugly, with a fake look. If the aesthetics are acceptable, another chunk of time will be spent on adjusting the occlusion. By this time the crown will probably have lost most of the glaze because of all the adjustments needed and the dentist will have to send it back to the lab for another glaze. One more appointment will be required for delivery. After all this effort and exercise in patience by both patient and dentist, a couple of years later the patient may come in with the porcelain fractured off. Moral of the story: a quality lab pays off in time saved, reduced crown remake expense and above all, peace of mind and the personal satisfaction of doing beautiful dentistry.

Crown Delivery

❖ The first step when delivering a crown is to check the contacts and adjust them if necessary. Sometimes the lab will make the crown a little wide on the interproximal surfaces, which prevents it from seating properly, leaving the margins open. Once the interproximal surfaces are adjusted and the crown sits properly, the next step is to check the margins. If there is a slight open margin, check the interproximal contacts again. While the assistant presses the crown against the tooth, pass the floss through the mesial and distal contacts. If you feel one or both are very tight, it is possible that there is still excess material on that surface which is preventing the crown from seating completely. Adjust the contact a little more and check the margins again. Occasionally, after further careful (in order not to open the interproximal contact) adjustment of the contact, the crown will slide in further, closing the margins.

Note: Whenever pressing down on a crown on the lower arch, the chin should be supported by whomever is doing the pressing. If is it the dentist who is pressing down, he/she can apply pressure on the crown with a thumb, while supporting the inferior portion of the mandible with the remaining four fingers of the same hand. This frees the other hand for work. If it is the assistant who is pressing down, he/she can apply pressure with the index finger of one hand while supporting the chin with the other hand. The reason for doing this is that it makes the procedure more comfortable for the patient by greatly reducing the pressure he would otherwise feel on his masticatory muscles and TMJ's.

❖ A way of determining where to grind when adjusting interproximal contacts: Place a thin, sturdy articulating paper— AccuFilm II (Parkell, Edgewood, NY) works well— vertically along the interproximal space. With the other hand insert the crown. The articulating paper is now between the adjacent tooth and the crown. Press down on the crown and pull on the articulating paper. This will mark the crown where it first touches the adjacent tooth. Adjust the crown by grinding slightly. After this initial adjustment, try flossing the interproximal space to determine if an adequate contact has been obtained. If not, repeat the process.

❖ After seating the crown, checking the margins, and before adjusting the occlusion, give the patient a hand mirror and ask him how he likes the crown. Imagine if, at this point, both the assistant and the dentist start saying how wonderful it looks, even if in reality the crown is not too wonderful. The patient may be swayed by these words into accepting the crown. Later, with time, he may conclude it is not aesthetic and become disappointed with the treatment. Therefore, let the patient have his say before you tell him what you think. If it is an anterior tooth or premolar and you see that its aesthetics can be improved, even if the patient says it is okay, explain to him what aspect you see can be improved and, if he agrees, make the change. This change can range from a simple shade adjustment to the fabrication of a new, more aesthetic crown. Some time may be lost and there may be an additional cost to you but, for years and years to come, the patient will have a more aesthetic smile.

❖   The reason to check the aesthetics before adjusting the occlusion is that, if the crown has to be remade due to inadequate aesthetics, you will not have wasted time doing the occlusal adjustment.

❖   When cementing the definitive crown, floss well, before the cement sets. Otherwise, it may be difficult and time consuming to remove hardened cement from the interproximal spaces. The way to do this is to have the assistant floss while you firmly hold the crown in place. A small knot in the floss will help to remove the soft cement. The assistant pushes the floss into the interproximal space, lets go of one end, and pulls the other end of the floss away from the mouth. The knot should be on the side that was released. This way it will go through the interproximal space removing the cement that is there. It is better that the assistant not simply pull the floss up through the interproximal contact since this may cause the crown to move ever so slightly. Any small movement of the crown at this point may affect the cementation process, weakening the bond between crown and tooth.

❖   If the tooth is vital and after having the temporary crown on for a few days there is no sensitivity to cold or any other discomfort, cement the final crown with a definitive cement.

❖   If the tooth is sensitive to cold after having had the temporary crown on for a few days, do not cement the final crown with a definitive cement since there is a possibility the tooth may end up needing RCT. Instead, cement the final crown with a mixture of temporary cement and Vaseline: three parts temporary cement to one part Vaseline. The Vaseline will make it easier to remove the crown if RCT becomes necessary. Give the tooth a few weeks. If the pain subsides, cement the crown with a definitive cement. If it persists or increases, remove the crown, do the RCT and cement the crown with a definitive cement. When the tooth in question is a premolar or an anterior tooth, consider placing a prefabricated post before definitively cementing the crown. The endodontic access will have further reduced and weakened the coronal tooth structure, and a post may strengthen it besides assisting in the retention of the core. Most of the literature does not support the view that a post may strengthen the remaining tooth structure in teeth that underwent RCT, but my clinical experience indicates that in maxillary premolars a post does prevent fracture of what coronal tooth structure is left. There is a clinical study that supports this view (for premolars in general).[12]

When the tooth being treated is a molar, there is usually no need for a post. Instead, one can fill the chamber and endodontic access with core build up material.[13] The bulk and shape of the pulp chamber provide retention and strength to the core build up material.

---

12 M. Ferrari, M.C. Cagidiaco, S. Grandini, M. De Sanctis, and C. Goracci. Post Placement Affects Survival of Endodontically Treated Premolars. *J Dent Res.* 2007 86(8):729-734.

13 Scotti N, et al. Is fracture resistance of endodontically treated mandibular molars restored with indirect onlay composite restorations influenced by fibre post insertion? *J Dent.* 2012 Oct; 40(10):814-20

Chapter 7

POST AND CORE

❖   When preparing the root canal for a post, it is recommended that 4 to 5 mm of root filling material be left to maintain the apical seal.[1] Consider having 5 mm of obturation material as your minimum when you prepare a post space. It is better for the patient that you take a more prudent approach and leave 5 mm of obturation material than that a lesser amount be left leading to infiltration, consequent development of an apical lesion and resultant failure of a costly treatment.

❖   If the root is short and leaving 5 mm of obturation material will result in a post with inadequate length, then the tooth is not a good candidate for a restoration. Consider extracting it and replacing it with an implant (or other prosthesis). A composite build-up with a short post is a temporary alternative to an extraction. It is important, in this case, to make it clear to the patient that the restoration will only be a temporary solution with the purpose of giving him some time to decide which treatment he wants for definitive tooth replacement. If the patient opts for the composite temporary, make sure to make an entry in his chart stating what you told him and his decision.

❖   Some guidelines for the length of the post:

1) Post length should ideally be 2/3 the length of the root.[2]

2) Post length should be at least equal to crown length.[3]

---

1 Gutmann J, Lovdahl P. *Problem Solving in Endodontics – Prevention Identification and Management*. Fifth Edition, Elsevier Pub. Pp.453.
2 Cheung W. A review of the management of endodontically treated teeth. Post, core and the final restoration. *J Am Dent Assoc*. 2005 May; 136 (5): 611-9.
3 Ibid

3) The post should extend to one-half the length of the root that is supported by bone.[4]

A short post increases the stress on the root and, therefore, increases the potential for a root fracture. It is common in daily practice to see a patient coming in with a debonded crown and post assembly or a fractured root with a resulting loose crown and post assembly. Upon inspection one finds, in most cases, that the post is very short.

❖   In molars, as stated in the previous chapter, the shape and large size of the pulp chamber usually allows for a strong, retentive core without the need for a post.

❖   Sometimes, when doing a composite core build up on a tooth with a deep interproximal box, gingival crevicular fluid will seep in between the matrix band and the gingival wall. The first step when this happens is to push the wooden wedge a little tighter into the interproximal space. If this does not stop the fluid penetration into the cavity, one can seal the space with a GI liner. With the Dycal placement instrument, place the GI liner along the matrix-gingival wall junction. This will prevent seepage and provide a dry field for the restoration of the tooth with resin composite. The margin with the unprotected GI liner will be covered by the crown, once it is placed, preventing the degradation of the material, which would otherwise occur if left exposed to the oral environment.

❖   When you are treatment planning for a post, examine the X-ray carefully. If the alveolar bone and PDL space surrounding the root have a normal aspect but the root canal obturation appears inadequate, such as if it is short (more than 2 mm from apex) or voids can be seen in the obturation material, retreat the canal prior to placing the post (or have it retreated by an endodontist). When the root canal obturation is inadequate, post preparation may disturb the apical seal and a lesion may develop after the post is cemented. The patient may return, two or three years after the post was placed, with pain on this tooth or, you may in a routine exam several years later see that an apical lesion has developed. When this happens, one is faced with the difficult decision

---

4 Ibid

of whether to redo all treatment, perform an apicoectomy, or extract the tooth and replace it with an implant.

❖ Consider always placing a post in a maxillary premolar that has had RCT. After the crown prep, even if most walls are intact, the remaining tooth structure in these teeth will usually be thin. The post seems to not only provide retention to the core but also to strengthen the tooth preventing fracture of tooth structure/core build up.[5] It is fairly common to see maxillary premolar crowns fracture off together with the underlying core when the RCT treated tooth either does not have a post or, if it does, it is of inadequate length.

❖ After initial obturation material removal with the Gates Glidden (GG) #2 drill, if you are not sure the preparation is at an adequate depth, take a PA X-ray to verify. When the tooth is under rubber dam isolation, one may leave the #2 GG drill in the canal for the X-ray in order to assist in visualizing the depth of the preparation.

❖ The minimum height for an adequate ferrule, to provide strength to the tooth-restoration unit, is 2 mm.[6] If there is 1 mm or less of coronal tooth structure along the whole circumference of the tooth, and the tooth is not a good candidate for a crown lengthening surgery, it is better not to do the post. If a post and crown are done, the greater probability is that within a short period of time, when the patient bites into an apple or other hard food, the post and crown assembly will come off or the root will fracture. The treatment of choice in this case is usually replacement with an implant supported crown. If the patient is unsure what to do, one may offer to place a prefabricated post and a chairside resin composite crown as a temporary until he is ready for a definitive treatment.

❖ Always try to perform the treatment under rubber dam isolation in order to prevent contamination of the canal space with saliva and consequent RCT failure at a later date. However, with cast posts this

5 M. Ferrari, M.C. Cagidiaco, S. Grandini, M. De Sanctis, and C. Goracci. Post Placement Affects Survival of Endodontically Treated Premolars. *J Dent Res.* 2007 86(8):729-734

6 Jotkowitz A, Samet N. Rethinking ferrule – a new approach to an old dilemma. *British Dental J.* 2010 Jul 209, 25 – 33.

may not always be practical, especially at the moment when one has to adjust the incisal or occlusal surface of the resin pattern. Whenever the tooth being worked on is not isolated with a rubber dam, the patient should remain with the mouth open (except when he has to bite in order to check if the resin pattern for a cast post is high) and the canal space should be kept free of saliva by isolation with cotton rolls. This, until the temporary crown and post are cemented in place and the canal is again sealed from the oral environment.

Flexi- Post

I learned in dental school to stay away from threaded posts because of the catastrophic root fractures that they often cause because of the strain they create on the root. It is good advice. However, there is a threaded post system that has the advantage of the retention produced by the threads without the disadvantage of the unfavorable stresses they can create.[7] The system is called Flexi-Post (Essential Dental Systems, South Hackensack, NJ).

Flexi-Post is a split shank, parallel-sided threaded post. Because of the split shank, the stresses of insertion are absorbed by the post, not the root, during placement. Therefore, unlike other threaded post systems, it does not cause root fractures if used properly.

❖   Flexi-Post works well for maxillary premolars.

❖   Usually, one post is sufficient for strengthening of the maxillary premolar and core retention. However, if both buccal and lingual prepared walls are thin and the tooth has two canals, one may consider placing one post in each canal. If you opt for this, make sure the canals do not converge at the crown. When such is the case, one post will be on the path of insertion of the other and you will only be able to place one of the two posts. While performing RCT, you may check if there is enough room for two posts by simultaneously placing a file, which fits

---

7 http://www.oralhealthgroup.com/features/endodontics-comparison-of-the-photoelastic-stress-properties-for-different-post-core-combinations/

snuggly, in each canal. If there are 2 or 3 mm of space between the two files at the occlusal level, there is room for two posts.

❖   For maxillary premolars, generally, the size 1 (red) Flexi-Post is used.

❖   Prepare the post space with Gates Glidden (GG) drills #2 and #4, and finish with the red Flexi-Post drill. It is important that the Flexi-Post drill penetrate the length of the post space created by the GG drills, or at least to 1 mm from length, for the post to go in smoothly and without excessive force.

A way to control the depth of the preparation is to place rubber stoppers on the GG drills at the length desired. Since the Flexi-Post drill is too thick for a rubber stopper, one can mark it at the desired length with a felt tip pen.

❖   Rinse the prepared post space with NaOCl canal irrigating solution and then make sure the canal is completely dry prior to post cementation. Use a good quality dual cure resin cement. Resin cement will bond with the resin composite core build up material creating a stronger restoration.

❖   When inserting the post, gently screw it in until you feel that it does not go any further. Then "turn back or unscrew" a quarter turn. This will reduce stress on the surrounding tooth structure.

❖   After the post has been inserted and prior to the hardening of the cement, fill the tooth with resin composite. Cure from the occlusal surface. After this initial cure, remove the matrix and cure the buccal and lingual surfaces through the tooth structure.

❖   When a tofflemire matrix is used during post cementation/core build up, and you plan to prepare for a crown in the same visit, you can place additional wedges at the coronal third of the interproximal surfaces giving these surfaces a "partially prepared form." That is, they will be 1 to 1.5 mm from the adjacent teeth making the final crown preparation easier.

❖   After finishing the crown preparation and further reducing the core build up material, again apply curing light to the occlusal surface and the mesial, distal, buccal and lingual surfaces. You may use two curing lights simultaneously, one at the buccal surface and one at the lingual surface and then (if there is room) one at the mesial and one at the distal. This will reduce the time needed to cure the composite.

Cast Post and Core

A cast post and core is a proven and successful restorative option.[8] It works well for maxillary incisors, mandibular premolars and all canines. It fits closely to the wide, tapering canal anatomy of these teeth and is a strong, cohesive unit.

❖   Remove the canal obturation material from the planed post space with Gates Glidden (GG) drills #2 and #4. Go to the length of the post space with both drills. If, after this, there remains obturation material on the walls of a wide, tapering canal, gently run a #4 GG or a #5 GG drill along its surfaces. This should remove the obturation material without removing excessive tooth structure.

❖   Occasionally, especially in older patients where the canal space is constricted, after removing the canal obturation material one is left with a narrow diameter post space at the cervical area. If the tooth is a maxillary central incisor, or a canine, which have wider roots and will require larger cores than maxillary lateral incisors, and which undergo stronger masticatory forces, consider enlarging the 2 to 3 mm coronal portion of the canal with GG drills #5 and #6. This will result in a stronger, slightly thicker post at its junction with the core.

❖   Before making the resin pattern of the post and core, prepare the coronal tooth structure for a crown. By crown prepping the tooth prior to the post impression, you will have an accurate knowledge of the

8 Marchi GM,et al. Effect of remaining dentine structure and thermal-mechanical aging on the fracture resistance of bovine roots with different post and core systems. *Int Endod J*. 2008 Nov; 41(11):969-76; Bacchi A, et al. Influence of post-thickness and material on the fracture strength of teeth with reduced coronal structure. *J Conserv Dent*. 2013 Mar-Apr; 16(2): 139–143. Creugers NH, et al. 5-year follow-up of a prospective clinical study on various types of core restorations. *Int J Prosthodont*. 2005 Jan-Feb; 18(1):34-9.

thickness of the remaining tooth walls. After the crown preparation, remove the portions of the remaining walls that are less than 1 mm in thickness. This is done because any tooth structure thinner than 1 mm may fracture off at post delivery or during function.[9]

Keep the margin supragingival in order to maintain dry the area you are working on. If the margin is placed subgingivally, gingival crevicular fluid and/or blood may seep into the canal contaminating it. At the following visit, after post cementation, the margins can be placed subgingivally if necessary.

❖ Occasionally, especially in teeth where the coronal tooth structure fractured off, the post space may be very round and the coronal tooth structure very flat. If this is the case, to prevent the post from rotating while in place and to facilitate cementation, a small groove may be placed in the coronal portion of the canal, creating a slot for the post. The portion of the post that fits into the groove will help to guide post placement and prevent post rotation.

❖ Irrigate with water to remove any loose obturation material from the post space prior to making the impression. Inject the water with mild to moderate force so that the water jet may dislodge obturation material that may be sticking to the canal walls. After this, irrigate with NaOCl gently so that there is no danger of it squirting beyond the canal opening. Have the assistant place a surgical suction right at the entrance to the canal while the canal is being irrigated.

❖ Coat the post space walls and coronal tooth structure with a thin layer of Vaseline prior to making the resin pattern. This will reduce the chances of it sticking to tooth structure (even with the use of Vaseline the resin can still stick to the canal walls; one must keep this in mind when doing this procedure).

❖ DuraLay resin (Reliance Dental Mfg., Alsip, IL) and DuraLay Plastic Pins (Reliance Dental Mfg., Alsip, IL), are good materials for the fabrication of a resin pattern of the post and core. The plastic pins are made specifically for post and core impression.

---

9 Jotkowitz A, Samet N. Rethinking ferrule – a new approach to an old dilemma. *British Dental J*. 2010 Jul; 209: 25 – 33.

❖   When making the resin pattern, cover the portion of the plastic pin that will go into the canal with DuraLay and insert it in the canal and hold it in place with one hand for 1 to 2 minutes. With the other hand, dip a cotton pellet in hot water and wet the DuraLay that has extruded from the canal. This is done to speed up the setting reaction. Once the acrylic starts to set (it starts to heat up), remove the plastic pin completely from the canal for a moment, inspect it, and reinsert it into the canal. A few voids in the resin pattern at this point are normal and expected. If the resin has been stripped from the pin, it is better to start over. After this initial complete removal and reinsertion, keep lifting and reinserting the plastic pin into the canal—a movement of 2 to 3 mm amplitude (do not remove it completely). This is done to prevent the DuraLay from sticking to the canal walls as it sets. If it sticks to the canal walls, it can be difficult to remove, and a fair amount of time will be spent in the process.

Once the DuraLay sets, remove the resin pattern from the canal and inspect it. If there are voids, add a thin, fluid layer of DuraLay to it and place it in the canal. While you wait the initial one to two minutes for the resin pattern to start to set, add DuraLay to the coronal portion of the plastic pin. Repeat the procedure of dabbing hot water on the DuraLay to speed up the setting reaction, and of removing and reinserting the plastic pin to prevent the resin pattern from binding to the canal walls. Once the DuraLay has set, check the resin pattern. The canal portion should be practically free of voids. With Sof-Lex (3M ESPE Dental, St. Paul, MN) discs or a crown prep bur, prepare the coronal portion of the resin pattern so that it looks exactly like what you desire the finished core to look like.

Initial adjustments of the resin pattern are more easily done outside of the patient's mouth. Final adjustments are done with the resin pattern seated in the tooth. Check the occlusion; make sure there is adequate clearance for the crown. By leaving the post and core with the final shape desired, less crown preparation time will be needed at the post delivery/final impression appointment.

❖   After finishing the impression and before adjusting the resin pattern, with an instrument, confirm that the length of the prepared canal space matches the length of the post impression. Place an instrument in the canal space (it can be an endodontic file or a periodontal probe), measure it and compare this with the length of the post (from apical end to where the core structure starts). If the post is short, a new resin pattern must be made.

❖ The temporary crown, in turn, may have a short post. A small cotton pellet can be pushed to the apex of the post space, and left there, prior to cementing the temporary crown and post. This will prevent temporary cement from flowing to that area, facilitating the removal of what little cement is in the canal at the following visit.

❖ Ask the dental laboratory to use a soft, yellow gold (gold type I). This will reduce crown preparation time (if any is necessary besides placing the margin subgingivally) because the bur will easily cut into the gold. It will also be aesthetic if an all-porcelain crown is placed, because yellow gold mimics dentin better than does a silver alloy.

❖ Send the resin pattern dry to the lab, there is no need to place it in water. When it is dry, there is a slight shrinkage of the acrylic.[10] This small reduction in size facilitates the gold post insertion into the canal at the following visit.

❖ At the post and core try-in/delivery, gently insert the post into the canal space. If there is some space between the core and tooth structure, the post is likely not sitting properly in the canal. Remove the post and core from the canal and inspect the post. With the use of a course Sof-Lex (3M ESPE Dental, St. Paul, MN) disc, grind any areas that are shiny, that is, that may be rubbing against the canal wall. If there are no shiny areas, give the post a general quick polish with the coarse Sof-Lex disc. Quite often this adjustment is enough for the unit to sit properly in the canal space. If it still does not fit, polish some more. If, after these adjustments, you see that the post is not going all the way into the canal space, or the post is now loose in the canal, the lab may have made a mistake somewhere along the line and you will have to make a new

---

10 Sabouhi M, Nosouhian S, Dakhilalian M, Davoudi A, Mehrad R. The effect of time and storage environment on dimensional changes of acrylic resin post patterns. *Open Dent J.* 2015 Jan 30; 9:87-90.

resin pattern. On the positive side, this rarely occurs, and, with a quality lab, it virtually never happens.

❖   Prior to the post and core cementation, take a PA with it in the canal to confirm that there is no space between the metal post and the obturation material.

❖   Remove any Vaseline or temporary cement which may be left in the canal prior to cementing the post. Wipe the canals with alcohol and then rinse with NaOCl. Wiping the canal walls can be done by wrapping cotton on an endodontic file, dipping it in alcohol and rubbing it against the canal walls.

❖   Place a retraction cord in the gingival sulcus prior to cementing the post. Use a Lentulo spiral drill to fill the canal with resin cement. Insert the post and leave in place the excess cement that will extrude from the canal. The excess cement will cover any gaps between the core and the tooth. You or the assistant must hold the post in place, applying mild pressure, for the time it takes the cement to set.

❖   Prepare the tooth for a crown. Very little preparation should be necessary at this point, most of it being done to place the margins where one desires. As one prepares the tooth for a crown, all excess cement is removed.

❖   The temporary crown which was used in the previous visit can be reused at this appointment. One just has to remove the acrylic post, hollow out the temporary and reline it on the prepared tooth.

Chapter 8

ROOT CANAL THERAPY

General Tips

❖ Do not do RCT without using a rubber dam. If the tooth can't be isolated with a rubber dam, it is a sign that crown lengthening surgery is necessary. If crown lengthening is contraindicated, then the tooth is a candidate for extraction and replacement with an implant. The rubber dam protects the patient from aspirating or swallowing small dental instruments such as files and makes the whole procedure much easier for the dentist by providing retraction of soft tissues and improving visibility. Also, and most importantly, it prevents contamination of the canal with saliva while the procedure is being performed.

❖ Consider using a light color rubber dam. It will reflect more light into the tooth and make it easier to see into the pulp chamber.

❖ Try to perform RCT, if indicated in the particular case you are treating, in one visit. It is better for the patient and for the office since it saves time.

❖ Call the patient at night after a RCT appointment in order to ask how he is doing.

❖ A couple of excellent books: *Problem Solving in Endodontics* by Gutmann and Lovdahl (easy to read from cover to cover); *Cohen's Pathways of the Pulp* by Hargreaves and Berman.

Materials

❖ **Gates Glidden drills (GG)** – These drills are very useful in enlarging the coronal third of a curved root canal, or the coronal half of a straight root canal, reducing the stress on the nickel titanium rotary files when the time comes to use them. Additionally, when a GG fractures, it generally breaks at the latch end rather than the bud end. In the rare instances when a fracture at the bud does occur, the clinician must generally utilize a surgical operating microscope and ultrasonics to facilitate removal.[1] If one cannot remove the separated instrument from the canal, one should refer to an endodontist at no charge to the patient. Note: I have had a few GG drills fracture at the latch end (one simply removes it from the canal with a cotton forceps) but never have I had a fracture at the bud end.

❖ **Round diamond bur size 2** - Use a small diameter round diamond bur, size #2 works well, to reach the pulp chamber. This avoids unnecessary tooth structure removal. Once the pulp chamber is reached, if the tooth has a large pulp chamber such as a molar, one can use a wider diameter bur to adjust the access. If it is an incisor the access can be adjusted with the same size bur used to reach the pulp chamber. When drilling through a porcelain or a PFM crown, consider always using a new bur. This will diminish the chances of the porcelain cracking. Before you start drilling through a crown, warn the patient that, "I have to drill through the crown in order to get to the canals. Sometimes, because of the drilling, the porcelain may fracture. The other option is to try to remove the crown, but the chances of the porcelain fracturing will be even greater, and/or the tooth itself may fracture because of the force that I will have to apply to it."

❖ **RC-Prep** (Premier Dental, Plymouth Meeting, PA) - For lubricating the endodontic files used in calcified canals.

❖ **Canal Irrigation Needles** - Use side delivery needles that are specifically designed for endodontic purposes to reduce the possibility of extrusion of NaOCl solution through the apex.

Prior to Starting RCT

❖ Remove all caries present and determine if the tooth is restorable. After determining if the tooth is restorable, explain to the patient the

---

1 Richard E. Mounce. Endodontic Instruments: A Primer on GG Drills. www.dentalcompare.com.

indicated treatment, its cost and prognosis. Explain that the alternative treatment option is extraction.

❖   Check the vitality—ice test and percussion test—of at least three teeth: the tooth in question and the adjacent teeth. The response to the tests on the adjacent teeth serves as a reference for the tests on the tooth in question. Also, although rarely, one may find that an adjacent tooth is necrotic. Note the findings in the chart.

❖   Check the vitality even if the suspect tooth has a radiolucency associated with its apex. Occasionally the tooth may be vital, the radiolucency being caused by an anatomical feature, such as the mental foramen, or by bone pathology not of pulpal origin, such as periapical cemental dysplasia.

❖   Check the periodontal condition of the tooth. If it is one of your active patients, the periodontal condition should be under control, that is, no active periodontal disease.   If it is a new patient with an endodontic emergency, he may also have active periodontal disease. When the tooth in question has mild to moderate attachment loss with a good prognosis from a periodontal standpoint, one may perform the RCT (to address the pain) before treating the periodontal condition. However, one must make sure the patient understands that he needs, not only RCT, but periodontal treatment as well. Explain to him that if the periodontal treatment is not performed, he may end up losing the tooth in question along with other teeth, because of progressive bone loss. After administering anesthesia for the RCT, and before isolating the tooth, scale and root plane its root surfaces. Use an ultrasonic scaler to gross debride its neighboring teeth. This should add only a few minutes to the total treatment time.

❖   When the tooth in question has more than 5 mm of attachment loss, active periodontal disease, and a poor prognosis, that is, you see that there are several missing teeth, the patient has poor oral hygiene, perhaps accompanied by a systemic condition such as diabetes, consider extraction. When a patient has poor oral hygiene and several missing teeth, usually this is an indication that he does not give much attention to his oral health. Any treatment performed in such an individual will have a poorer prognosis than on a person who takes care of his teeth. Hence the indication for an extraction. Offer to refer the patient to a periodontist prior to extracting the tooth and make a notation in the chart that you have done so. If the above patient is interested in saving the tooth, you can alleviate the pain in most cases of irreversible pulpitis by doing a pulpotomy/pulpectomy, placing a cotton pellet with eugenol in the pulp chamber and sealing it with a temporary restoration.[2] From a practical point of view, one can charge the patient for a sedative filling in addition to the X-rays and emergency exam. Before continuing with the treatment, however, refer the patient to a periodontist for evaluation. This so that the patient does not incur the expense of a root canal needlessly. Once the periodontist has determined that the tooth can be maintained and has given the go ahead for treatment, the RCT can be finished. In a situation like this it is very important to educate the patient about periodontal disease and about the importance of trying to maintain his teeth. An educated patient will likely be more motivated to finish his treatment (endo, perio, restorative) and to take proper care of his teeth.

❖ In an anterior tooth, explain to the patient that the shade of the coronal tooth structure may undergo some change after RCT.

❖ For posterior teeth have a BW and a PA X-ray taken. The BW will give you a more accurate idea of the shape of the pulp chamber. The PA will give you an idea of: (1) apical condition; (2) shape of roots and canals; (3) degree of calcification of canals.

Anesthesia

❖ Give profound anesthesia—Septocaine with epinephrine 1:100,000 is very effective.[3] In a healthy patient usually two carpules, whether infiltrative or block, will obtain profound anesthesia. The exception to

2 McDougal R, et al. Success of an alternative for interim management of irreversible pulpitis. *J Am Dent Assoc*. 2004 Dec; 135 (12): 1707-12.
3 Rogers B, et al. Efficacy of Articaine versus Lidocaine as a Supplemental Buccal Infiltration in Mandibular Molars with Irreversible Pulpitis: A Prospective, Randomized, Double-blind Study. *J Endod* 2014 Jun; 40 (6): 753–758.

this is irreversible pulpitis in mandibular posterior teeth (especially molars).[4]

❖   When a molar in the lower arch has irreversible pulpitis, often the inferior alveolar nerve block does not result in complete anesthesia, it only lessens the pain. In these cases, consider also administering an intraosseous injection of anesthetic after administering the mandibular block and obtaining lip numbness, but before starting to drill the tooth.[5] On the other hand, you may first test the degree of numbness by drilling the tooth and only then, if the patient feels pain, administer the intraosseous anesthesia. The problem with this approach is that, in an anxious patient, once he feels pain, his stress level will likely go up and the treatment from then on can become tense and difficult.

❖   Some points about intraosseous anesthesia:

1) It is better not to tell the patient that you are going to, "give an intraosseous anesthesia." This sounds painful and will likely cause him some apprehension. He may ask what intraosseous anesthesia is and really get stressed when part of your explanation is that a hole will be drilled in the bone. When giving a mandibular block one does not describe it in detail such as, "I am going to puncture the mucosa with a needle, it will likely penetrate through muscle, then it will probably hit the bone and I will deposit the anesthetic right next to the nerve." One normally just says something like, "You are going to feel a little pinch, sorry about that." In the same way, when administering intraosseous anesthesia one can just say: "I am going to give a little more anesthesia," and go about the business of administering the intraosseous anesthesia.

2) Before drilling, warn the patient, "You may feel some vibration." Before injecting the solution, warn the patient that, "You may feel your

---

4 Claffey E, et al. Anesthetic efficacy of articaine for inferior alveolar nerve blocks in patients with irreversible pulpitis. *J Endod*. 2004 Aug; 30(8): 568-71.
5 Nusstein J, et al. Anesthetic efficacy of the supplemental intraosseous injection of 2% lidocaine with 1:100,000 epinephrine in irreversible pulpitis. *J Endod*. 1998 Jul;24(7):487-91; Reisman D, Reader A, Nist R, Beck M, Weaver J. Anesthetic efficacy of the supplemental intraosseous injection of 3% mepivacaine in irreversible pulpitis. *Oral Surg Oral Med Oral Pathol Oral Radiol Endod*. 1997 Dec; 84(6):676-82.

heart beating a little faster, but this is normal, and the sensation subsides in a couple of minutes."

3) X-tip system (Dentsply, York, PA) works very well because it leaves a guide sleeve through the cortical plate into which one can insert the needle. This makes finding the drilled hole a nonissue. In intraosseous anesthesia systems that drill into bone but do not leave a guide, it can be difficult to find the drilled hole with the injection needle.

4) If, while injecting, there is a backflow of anesthetic into the oral cavity, the tooth will likely not be anesthetized. Consider drilling another hole into the cortical bone and trying again.

5) The onset of the anesthesia is immediate.

6) With the X-tip system you may drill the hole in the mucosa or the attached gingiva.

An excellent guide on intraosseous anesthesia is the online article: American Association of Endodontists. Endodontics: Colleagues for excellence. "Intraosseus Anesthesia." Winter 2009.[6]

❖   As a last resort, when the patient is feeling pain, there is intrapulpal anesthesia. It always works but is very painful.

❖   For maxillary molars, in addition to the infiltrative anesthesia administered on the buccal, consider administering also approximately 1/3 of a cartridge (0.6 ml) in the palate, at the area of the apex of the palatal root. This is done as a preventive measure because, occasionally, perhaps due to the distance of the apex of the palatal root to the buccal vestibule, the infiltrative anesthesia administered solely on the buccal may not completely numb the tooth.

Endodontic Access

❖   Before starting the endodontic access preparation, take a good look at the X-ray. In posterior teeth, by looking at the BW X-ray you will have an idea of the distance from the occlusal surface to the roof of the pulp

---

6 https://www.aae.org/uploadedfiles/publications_and_research/
endodontics_colleagues_for_excellence_newsletter/winter2009_bonusmaterialf.pdf

chamber. If you use digital X-rays, the software can easily measure this distance. If you use conventional film, measure the distance with a ruler. This information will allow you to know how many mm the bur must penetrate tooth structure in order to reach the pulp chamber. While drilling, use magnification and bright illumination so that you can see well. Go about the endodontic access very calmly. Check often the pulpal wall of the access preparation. These factors together will keep you from reaching the floor of the pulp and perforating it.

❖ If you see that it will be a difficult endodontic access preparation due to an abnormal tooth inclination, do the endodontic access preparation without the rubber dam. By being able to see the tooth that is being treated in comparison with the other teeth while you drill, you will have a much better idea of the tooth's long axis inclination, greatly reducing the chances of a perforation or unnecessary removal of healthy tooth structure.

❖ If upon looking at the BW X-ray, you see that the pulp chamber in a posterior tooth is very calcified, start the endodontic access at the center of the occlusal surface and aim the bur at the largest canal. Thus, in a lower molar the bur will be aimed at the distal canal; in a maxillary molar the bur will be aimed at the palatal canal. Both these canals are normally wider than the other canals and are usually aligned with the midline of their respective wall (distal canal: middle of distal wall; palatal canal: middle of palatal wall). This reduces the chances of an inadvertent perforation of the pulp chamber floor.

❖ In a posterior tooth if, inadvertently, a small perforation is drilled on the floor of the pulp chamber while one is trying to access the canal, the RCT may be finished and, afterwards, ProRoot MTA (Dentsply, York, PA) used to repair the perforation.[7] First obtain hemostasis, then place GI liner over the perforation to protect the area. Finish the RCT. When done, remove the GI liner and cover the perforation with MTA. It is important to let the patient know a perforation has occurred, make

7 Silveira C, et al. Repair of furcal perforation with mineral trioxide aggregate: long-term follow-up of 2 cases. *J Can Dent Assoc.* 2008 Oct; 74(8):729-33.

the appropriate entry in the chart and do follow up exams in order to monitor healing progress.

❖   If the tooth has a crown and the plan is to replace it, consider removing the crown prior to starting the RCT. This will allow much more light to penetrate the tooth than when the crown is in place, and will consequently greatly improve visibility of the pulp chamber and canal entrances. This guideline applies especially for molars. WAMkey (WAM, France) is a very good crown and bridge remover. It is quick to use, atraumatic (and not scary to either patient or dentist) and allows you to reuse the crown as a temporary. The downside is that one has to drill a small whole in the buccal surface of the crown in order to insert the instrument. But if the plan is to make a new crown, this should not be   an   issue.   There   are   several   videos   available   at http://www.wamkey.com that show how it is used. Occasionally, when using the WAMkey, if the crown has good retention, the porcelain on the occlusal may fracture off and the metal below it bend. This is the reason why it may be safer to use it only on crowns which one plans to replace.

❖   After the endodontic access, rubber dam isolation and before exploring the canals, irrigate the pulp chamber with NaOCl to remove debris.

❖   When preparing the endodontic access, and later when looking for the canal entrances, keep in mind that there is a range of number of root canals that any given tooth can have. Mandibular molars, for example, can have as little as one canal and as much as more than four canals.

Measuring the Canal(s) - Using the Apex Locator

❖   Measure the apparent length of the tooth in the X-ray image and place the rubber stopper on the files you will use to explore the canals at the same length. While exploring the canal, measure the true working length with the apex locator.

❖   An additional method of determining the working length is to take a PA with a #15 K file in the canal and measure the distance from the tip of the file to the radiographic apex of the root. However, this is not the most reliable method since the apical foramen may be short of the radiographic apex.

❖ Use the apex locator often during the canal preparation phase in order to confirm that the canal is not being instrumented beyond or short of working length.

❖ Normally, the apex locator works well, independently of whether the canal is dry or wet. Occasionally, however, one may not get clear readings. When this is the case, try drying the canal before using the apex locator. Also, if the readings are not clear, make sure the tooth is well isolated, with no saliva seeping in.

❖ When the tooth being treated has a metal or PFM crown, the apex locator normally does not give clear readings if the file is touching the metal.

❖ One should have the tooth being worked on and the apex locator display screen almost in the same field of view so that, while one is instrumenting, with just a shift of the eyes, one can look from tooth to display screen and back to tooth. It helps also to have the alarm sound on. The alarm sounds as the file approaches the apex and the tone changes once it is reached.

Exploring the Canal(s)

❖ For anterior teeth and mandibular premolars, usually a #15 K file can be used to explore the canal and will comfortably reach the apex. In molars and, occasionally, maxillary premolars, a #10 K file will normally reach the apex more easily than the #15 K file.

❖ Exploring molar canals: Curve the tip of the #10 K file that will be used to explore the canals. Do not rotate the file 360 degrees in the canal since this may cause it to break. Instead, do quarter turns as you try to gain depth. Attach the apex locator file holder to the file as it penetrates close to the apparent working length. Once WL is reached, with the file holder or a cotton forceps push the rubber stopper to the reference point on the tooth. Remove the file from the canal, measure the WL, reinsert it and instrument the canal. If you feel the file curving severely as it penetrates a canal (the file will stiffen and press against a wall instead of being centered in the canal), with a small round bur remove the dentin at the area where the file presses as it exits the canal. By removing this area of dentin, a more direct path of insertion will be created and there will be less file bending and less chance of file breakage.

In the great majority of cases the #10 K file will reach WL. If, however, it does not go to WL, switch to a #8 K file. If the #8 K file has not reached WL, but you feel you are 3 mm from the apex at the most, do not become anxious and force the file down. By forcing the file, you may create a ledge or the file may break. As you enlarge the cervical portion of the canal, files will usually gradually reach WL.

If both #8 and #10 K files are farther than 3 millimeters from the apex, it is better to stop the treatment at this point and refer the patient to an endodontist. It is important to stop here to avoid creating a ledge, which will make it more difficult for the endodontist to reach working length.

Canal Preparation - General Tips

❖   When using the rotary files, do so with the apex locator file holder attached to the file. This, in addition to the rubber stopper set at the desired length, will allow you to instrument exactly at working length, and not beyond it. Note: Always clip the file holder to the upper part of file shaft, near the head of the contra-angle.

❖   In straight canals, after instrumenting with a #20 K file prepare the cervical 5 mm to 6 mm of canal space with GG drill #2 followed by GG drill #4. This step speeds up canal preparation and prevents binding of the rotary files to the cervical portion of the canal. Irrigate with NaOCl after each drill use.

❖   When the canal is calcified, it seems to me that lubricating the hand files used during exploration and initial shaping with a gel type lubricant, such as RC-prep (Premier Dental Products, Plymouth Meeting, PA), facilitates penetration of the files into the canal. Studies show, however, that gel type lubricant increase the torque on rotary files.[8] Therefore, one should avoid using gel type lubricants with rotary files.

❖   These two guidelines greatly help to prevent file breakage:

1) Never apply more than a slight force to the rotary files.

2) Always use a new set of rotary files for each tooth treated.

❖   Irrigate well after each file use. When irrigating, do not get closer to the apex than 3 mm with the irrigation needle tip and do not irrigate with force. The irrigation needle should not wedge into the canal so that there is room for a backflow of solution as you apply light pressure to the syringe. If NaOCl extrudes beyond the apex, the patient will immediately feel pain. Depending on the amount of solution extruded, there will be almost instant swelling in addition to the severe pain. A guide   on   NaOCl   extrusion   accidents   can   be   found   at http://healthma.bizland.com/rotary/hyochorite%20in%20endo.pdf. This article outlines how to prevent these accidents from happening and how to treat them if they do occur.

❖   If a ledge is inadvertently created in the canal, bend the tip of a #10 K file in the same direction of the mark on the rubber stopper (the reason for this is that once the file is in the canal, past the ledge, by looking at the notch in the rubber stopper you will know in which direction the ledge is situated). Gently insert the file in the canal and do quarter turns until you feel it go past the ledge. Make a mental note of the direction to which the mark on the rubber stopper was pointing when the file went past the ledge. This will tell you to which direction the curvature in the other files you will use must be pointing to go past the ledge. Once the initial file goes past the ledge, do not remove it immediately. Instead, penetrate as deep as you can and instrument, applying pressure against the ledge. If you remove the file from the canal before instrumenting against the ledge, it may be difficult to go past it again. After filing against the ledge, remove the file. Work yourself up to a #20 or #25 K file and follow this with the rotary files.

---

8 Peters O, Boessler C, Zehnder M. Effect of liquid and paste-type lubricants on torque values during simulated rotary root canal instrumentation. *Int Endod J*. 2005 Apr; 38(4):223-9.

❖   Have a gauze sponge drenched in alcohol on the instrument tray. Each time a file (whether handheld or rotary) is taken out of the canal, have the assistant wipe it with the gauze to remove any debris in its flutes. The file will cut better when it is used again if its grooves are free of particles.

❖   The root canal in anterior teeth and mandibular premolars can often be quickly instrumented. If you have finished instrumenting the canal in a short period of time, consider leaving the canal drenched in NaOCl for 10 minutes or so, before obturating.

After instrumenting, remove the smear layer with 17% EDTA aqueous solution and then flush the canal with 5% NaOCl. Leave the canal filled with the solution. After 5 minutes, again irrigate with NaOCl leaving it drenched for another 5 minutes. This will better disinfect the canal than if it is obturated promptly after a quick instrumentation.[9] The reason for removing the smear layer with the EDTA solution is that this will allow for a more thorough disinfection of the canal and penetration of the sealer into the dentinal tubules.[10]

❖   Once finished with the canal preparation, dry gently. Do not push the paper point abruptly and quickly into the canal because this may push NaOCl through the apex causing pain.

❖   DO NOT spray air into the canal space since this may cause air emphysema. If it occurs, the patient will have a swollen face for a few days, and one will have to consider prescribing him antibiotics in order to prevent an infection. It will be an unpleasant and potentially dangerous situation that could have been easily avoided by drying the pulp chamber with cotton pellets instead of an air spray.

❖   Irrigating needles must be always calibrated with a rubber stopper in order to prevent inserting them too deeply, or, too close to the apex.

❖   It is better not to leave NaOCl in a plastic syringe with a rubber plunger tip for more than a couple of hours. If NaOCl is left for a longer

9 Deivanayagam Kandaswamy and Nagendrababu Venkateshbabu. Root canal irrigants. *J Conserv Dent*. 2010 Oct-Dec; 13(4): 256–264.
10 Hargraves K, Cohen S. Cohen's *Pathways of the Pulp*. Tenth Edition. Elsevier Publishing; 2011. Pp 356 - 357

period in the syringe, it will start to degrade the rubber plunger tip and be contaminated with small rubber particles.

Molar Canal Preparation Tips

❖ After the #8 (if necessary) and #10 K files, instrument with #15 and #20. All to WL, if possible. If WL was not reached with the #8 file, work yourself up to a #20 regardless, carefully so as not to over instrument and create a ledge close to the apex. The main goal is to obtain canal patency up to the apical third of the canal.

❖ After using the #20 K file, enlarge the entrance to the canal with GG drills #2 to #4. This will widen the entrance to the canal and allow the files to go in with less curvature. At this point, do not penetrate more than 2 mm into the canal with each GG drill to avoid creating a ledge.

When WL has been reached: instrument canal with #25K file.

When WL has not been reached: instrument again with #15 K file. Occasionally, after enlarging the entrance to the canal, the file will go to WL. If there is no gain in depth, go to #25 K file.

❖ After #25, use again the #2 GG drill. This time, drill up to 5 or 6 mm into the canal. Do not force the drill and do not hold it at a certain depth for more than an instant. As soon as you feel that the drill is not gaining depth or that there is an increase in resistance, remove it to avoid creating a ledge. If you see on the X-ray that there is a curve in the canal, drill 2 mm short of it. This also to avoid creating a ledge.

❖ Finish the preparation with rotary files. With the use of rotary files, WL should be reached if the canal preparation is still 1 to 2 mm short.

Obturation

❖ Gutta-percha cones should go to WL and bind at the apex. Prior to obturation, a PA should be taken with the master cone in place to confirm that it is at the desired length in the canal. There are several different obturation systems available. A guideline is to choose a system that studies show has good results, and use always this same system in order for you to become comfortable and quick in its use.

Temporary Restoration

❖ When placing a temporary restoration in a tooth in which you just finished the RCT (and in a tooth undergoing RCT), keep in mind that the restoration must provide adequate seal. If there is coronal leakage while the tooth is temporized, there will be bacterial contamination and an increased probability of RCT failure. If you feel the patient may take more than a few days to come back for the definitive restoration (or to finish the RCT), restore the endo access with glass ionomer cement. This will improve the chances of the pulp chamber remaining sealed until the patient returns.[11] Independently of which material is used, the temporary restoration should be at least 4 to 5 mm thick.[12]

❖ In molars, when possible, when done with the root canal and after removing all obturation material from the pulp chamber, fill it with the resin composite core build up material. That is, place the definitive material in the pulp chamber, no cotton pellet necessary. This procedure takes only a few minutes to be done since the tooth is under rubber dam isolation. The bonded restoration provides the best seal the tooth can have. In this way, if the patient delays in coming back for the definitive restoration, the canals are sealed and protected from coronal infiltration and, also, the tooth is strengthened by the bonded core material.

❖ Sometimes, usually due to financial reasons, the patient who underwent a molar RCT wants to wait an indefinite period to have a crown placed. When this is the case, the core build up must then be as good as a definitive composite, with adequately shaped interproximal walls and occlusal anatomy, and with physical properties that will allow it to withstand occlusal function. Therefore, even though the core material has already been placed, schedule an appointment to redo the

11 Barthel CR, et al. Leakage in roots coronally sealed with different temporary fillings. *J Endod.* 1999 Nov; 25(11): 731-4.
12 Hargraves K, Cohen S. *Cohen's Pathways of the Pulp.* Tenth Edition. Elsevier Publishing; 2011. Pp 272

coronal portion of the restoration. At this visit remove a 2 to 3 mm layer of composite core build up material from any external surface where it is present and consider also removing any remaining cusps to reduce the chances of tooth fracture. Restore with the composite restorative material you normally use for posterior teeth.

Retreatment

❖   My advice is not to retreat molars. Not even to try. It is best to refer the patient to an endodontist. Quite commonly, a molar that has an inadequate RCT will have ledges on the canal walls, blocked canals or even perforations. If you attempt to retreat, it is very unlikely you will be able to solve these problems and the responsibility for them will now be yours.

Chapter 9

PERIODONTAL TREATMENT

❖ Educate the patient. The success of your treatment depends on the patient being motivated to maintain excellent oral hygiene and to come in for regular periodontal maintenance cleanings.[1] You can say something like, "Studies show that among persons who have finished treatment for periodontal disease, those who have maintenance cleanings every 3 months, over a period of time lose less bone and teeth than those who don't." As you explain about bone loss, show an FMX of a healthy dentition and one of a case with advanced bone loss. Illustrate your explanations with drawings and pictures. Teach the patient about the relationship between periodontitis and systemic conditions such as diabetes, cardiovascular disease, and chronic obstructive pulmonary disease.

❖ If the patient smokes, without being overbearing, explain to him the effects of smoking on the periodontal tissues. You can say, "Smoking has an association with periodontal disease. Studies show that smokers have four times the chance of having periodontitis in comparison to nonsmokers.[2] However, once the person quits, with time, he will again develop some resistance to periodontal disease.[3] Also, in persons with periodontal disease, the ones who smoke will lose bone faster than the nonsmokers.[4] I know it is not easy to quit but maybe

---

1 Checchi L, et al. Retrospective study of tooth loss in 92 treated periodontal patients. *J Clin Periodontol*. 2002 Jul; 29(7): 651-6. Tsami A, et al. Parameters affecting tooth loss during periodontal maintenance in a Greek population. *J Am Dent Assoc*. 2009 Sep; 140(9): 1100-7.
2 Haber J, et al. Evidence for cigarette smoking as a major risk factor for periodontitis. *J Periodontology*. 1993; 64: 16
3 d'Fiorini T, et al. Is there a positive effect of smoking cessation on periodontal health? A systematic review. *J Periodontology*. 2014 Jan; 85(1): 83-91.
4 Bolin A, et al. The effect of changed smoking habits on marginal alveolar bone loss. A longitudinal study. *Swed. Dent J*. 1993; 17(5): 211-6.

now is a good time to give it a try." Refer the patient to a smoking cessation program if he is interested.

❖ It has been stipulated that the total surface area of infected and inflamed pocket epithelium in a patient with generalized moderate periodontitis and a full complement of teeth is roughly equivalent to the size of the palm of his hand. This comparison can be used to educate the patient and help him visualize the urgency and necessity of obtaining treatment.[5]

❖ When a patient presents with active chronic generalized periodontal disease, first perform gross debridement, and give oral hygiene instruction. At the following visits, perform scaling and root planning (SC and RP). The reason for this is that the gross debridement and improved OH will promote initial gingival healing causing the marginal gingiva to shrink and become less susceptible to bleeding. These two factors will make it easier for the hygienist to see the exposed portion of the roots and perform a thorough SC and RP at the next visit.

❖ If at the first periodontal maintenance prophylaxis (3 months after SC and RP has been completed) the patient presents with bleeding upon probing or pockets with probing depths of 6 mm or more, and you do not have the training to perform periodontal surgery, consider referring him to a periodontist. If the patient presents with no bleeding upon probing, healthy gingiva and pockets of 5 mm or less, keep him on a 3 month periodontal maintenance recall. As mentioned above, studies show that this recall regimen prevents bone loss.

❖ If, prior to treatment, the BW X-rays show calculus at the interproximal surfaces, have the hygienist take another BW when he/she has finished scaling and root planning the area, to confirm that the interproximal calculus has been removed. Teach him/her to do this on his/her own, without your having to ask. He/She must do this in addition to checking the scaled root surfaces with an explorer for the presence of remaining calculus.

---

5 Page, R. The pathobiology of periodontal diseases may affect systemic diseases: inversion of a paradigm. *Ann Periodontol.* 1998 Jul;3(1): 108-20.

❖   Consider performing crown lengthening surgeries only if you have advanced training. When it comes to crown lengthening surgery on anterior teeth, it may be prudent to always refer the patient to a periodontist. The dark triangle created by the loss of an interdental papilla, or an exposed cemento-enamel junction created by post-surgical gingival shrinkage, can be very unaesthetic. The patient may, understandably, become displeased with the outcome of the procedure. One may end up losing him as a patient and probably all his family and friends as well.

❖   Pericoronitis associated with partially erupted wisdom teeth is a condition that one often encounters in clinical practice. There usually is spontaneous, moderate to severe pain. The gingiva partially covering the distal portion of the tooth will be erythematous, swollen and will be painful to the touch. When the infection is localized, which is how it presents in most cases, with the use of a monoject syringe, gently irrigate around the crown with chlorhexidine or a warm saline solution. Gently debride the area with a hand or ultrasonic scaler. Have the patient rinse with 3% hydrogen peroxide every 2 hours for the first day, holding the medication over the infected area for 30 seconds or so, and whenever symptoms develop from thereon. When the acute infection has subsided, the tooth may be extracted, if this is the indicated treatment. The reason not to remove the tooth at the emergency visit is that, occasionally, a wisdom tooth extraction may require flap reflection and osteotomy. It is safer to perform these procedures when there is no acute infection present.[6]

When, in addition to the acute local infection, there is lymphadenopathy, trismus, fever, or diffuse swelling of the soft tissues, prescribe antibiotics besides debriding the area.

---

6 Cawson R, Odell E. *Cawson's Essentials of Oral Pathology and Oral Medicine*. 8th Edition. Elsevier Publishing; 2008. pg 92.

Chapter 10

EXTRACTION

Tooth Factors to be Considered Prior to an Extraction

❖   Sometimes an emergency patient will present with pain in a tooth that is restoratively in good condition, needing perhaps only a small restoration or, occasionally, no restoration at all (the tooth may already have a crown or a filling that is in good condition), the pain being caused by an inflamed or necrotic pulp and the tooth requiring RCT. If this patient cannot afford the RCT but is interested in maintaining the tooth, consider referring him to a school or clinic where he can have the treatment done for free or at low price. Take the steps to relieve his discomfort prior to dismissing him. It is important in a case like this, to make sure the patient understands that you are providing him with temporary relief and that the pain can return anytime, in a few days or a few weeks, if RCT is not done. In addition, explain that if RCT is not done, a painful abscess and swelling of the face will likely occur. Make notations in the chart of what you told the patient and what the patient said to you.

An example of the above would be an emergency patient with a maxillary central incisor with irreversible pulpitis. Most people do not want to lose any teeth, much less a maxillary central incisor. But not all can afford the RCT. In a few minutes you can do a pulpectomy, place a cotton pellet with eugenol in the pulp chamber and place a temporary restoration.[1] Prior to starting, explain to the patient that, "This tooth needs either RCT or an extraction. Since you cannot afford the RCT at present an alternative to extracting this tooth is to remove the nerve (pulp) to relieve the pain. But this is only a temporary treatment. You must go as soon as possible to (say the name of the dental clinic—

---

1 McDougal R, Delano E, Caplan D, Sigurdsson A, Trope M. Success of an alternative for interim management of irreversible pulpitis. *J Am Dent Assoc.* 2004 Dec; 135 (12): 1707-12.

provide patient with address and phone number) in order to have the RCT done. If you don't go, the tooth can start hurting severely again in a few days. Also, if the RCT is not done, an abscess may develop, and you will have severe pain and a swollen face."

❖ If an anterior tooth has advanced periodontal disease, is asymptomatic, and has indication for extraction, explain clearly to the patient that the tooth must be extracted and what the replacement options are. If the patient does not want to extract the tooth or is unsure, do not insist on performing the procedure. Instead, refer the patient to another dentist for a second opinion. If you put yourself in the patient's shoes and imagine losing a front tooth, it will be easier to understand his reluctance. The second opinion will help him be at peace with the treatment needed.

❖ Make it a point to always replace an anterior tooth at the time of extraction. Therefore, before extracting an anterior tooth, plan with the patient how it will be replaced. (For posterior teeth it suffices to explain to the patient the different tooth replacement alternatives prior to extracting the tooth.) Some of the ways to temporarily replace an anterior tooth are: (1) a lab made flipper; (2) a flipper made in office; (3) sectioning off the crown of the tooth to be extracted and bonding it to the adjacent teeth (if the coronal tooth structure is in good condition such as may happen in advanced periodontal disease); (4) bonding a composite crown, made in office, to the adjacent teeth. In all these options it is important to emphasize to the patient that the treatment is temporary, can fail at any moment, and that he must avoid cutting foods with his front teeth (regarding the flippers, ideally the patient should take them off to eat).

❖ Always have a quality, recent, periapical X-ray of the tooth being extracted. One that shows at least a few millimeters of bone beyond the root tips. The image should be clear, not blurry. Sometimes the tube head is moving while the assistant, in a hurry, takes the X-ray, or the patient moves, resulting in a blurry image. Teach the assistant what is an acceptable image so that, if the X-ray is inadequate, he/she can retake it before you walk into the operatory. This saves time since, after coming into the operatory and looking at the X-ray, you don't have to ask the assistant to repeat it, leave again and wait until the new one is ready.

❖ As mentioned on page 3, an excellent book to have in the dental office to serve as a reference guide regarding the treatment of medically compromised patients is: *page,* by Donald A. Falace and James W. Little. Elsevier Publishing.

Systemic Factors and Extractions

❖ Check the medical history carefully. If the patient is an older person, checks the "no" boxes for all questions in the medical questionnaire (no high blood pressure, no diabetes…), and tells you not to worry, that everything is fine, become suspicious (worry!). Ask specifically if he takes blood thinners, high blood pressure meds, hypoglycemic agents, etc. Call his physician to ascertain that he is healthy. Often these patients mean no harm to themselves or to you. They may have one or more systemic conditions but are just "old school" and want to seem tough. They believe that no adverse effects can happen from a "simple" dental treatment.

❖ Have the assistant measure the patient's blood pressure (BP) before every extraction you perform. This is a service you do to the patient since you may catch an undiagnosed high blood pressure (HBP). Make a notation in the chart of the findings.

❖ If the diastolic BP is over 110 or if the systolic BP is over 170 do not perform an extraction. In both cases refer the patient to his physician and explain to him that his HBP must be addressed before the extraction can be done. If the extraction is done while the BP is high a hemorrhage may occur.[2]

❖ Whenever the patient is taking blood thinners or if you are the least bit unsure that patient is a good candidate for an extraction due to a systemic condition or a medication he takes, call his physician and obtain his consent prior to doing the extraction. Make a notation in the

---

2 Little F, Falace D, Miller C, Rhodus N. *Dental Management of the Medically Compromised Patient.* Eighth Edition. Elsevier Publishing; 2013, p 46.

chart that you have done so and of what the physician said. You can also have the physician's office fax you his instructions and consent.

❖   In diabetic patients, test the blood glucose level before starting the procedure. Glucometers are available for sale at most drugstores. If the blood glucose level (whether fasting or postprandial) is over 200 mg/dL, defer treatment and refer the patient to his physician. If the extraction is done before the glucose level is normalized, a severe post operatory infection may occur.[3]

❖   Watch out for uncontrolled diabetes. When the patient has complications arising from uncontrolled diabetes, such as renal or heart disease, consult with his physician prior to performing an extraction.

❖   Never do an extraction on a hemophiliac. Refer to an oral surgeon. I know this is obvious, but it does not hurt to mention it.

❖   If the patient has had radiation therapy of the head and neck region and needs an extraction, refer to an oral surgeon. Osteoradionecrosis may occur as a result of an extraction in irradiated bone. The oral surgeon is better prepared to take the necessary steps to diminish the probability of this occurring and to treat it if it does occur.

❖   When the patient takes Bisphosphonates, the prudent course is to refer him to an oral surgeon.[4]

❖   If the patient automedicated with an antibiotic, make sure to write in the chart: "Patient automedicated with antibiotic." Teach the patient not to do so anymore. Explain to him the consequences of doing so. When the patient frequently automedicates with antibiotics, a severe infection, difficult to treat, may develop after an extraction.

❖   When there is facial cellulitis associated with a tooth that will not be extracted in the same visit, or will not be extracted at all, in addition to prescribing antibiotics, an incision and drainage will help to control the infection. This procedure creates a pathway for pus and exudate

---

3 Ibid, p. 235.
4 Guidelines on the management of these patients can be found at
https://lexi.com/individuals/ dentistry/newsletters.jsp?id=december_11.

drainage, provides immediate pain relief, and facilitates blood flow to the area increasing the efficacy of the antibiotic.[5]

❖   If you see that the extraction may be difficult, requiring osteotomy, and there is an acute infection with facial cellulitis present, get the infection under control first by performing an incision and drainage and prescribing antibiotics. After three or four days of antibiotic therapy, if there is no swelling, the infection should be under control, and it should be safe to do the extraction. The problem with doing a complicated extraction with osteotomy in the presence of an acute infection, is that there is a possibility that osteomyelitis may develop.

Call the patient on the first night after seeing him, in order to ask how he is doing. If the swelling has not diminished by the following day after incision, drainage, and commencement of antibiotic therapy, refer him to an oral surgeon.

Another option for this case is to immediately refer the patient to an oral surgeon who may perform the incision and drainage, and the extraction, in a hospital setting.

Keep in mind, when performing an incision and drainage, that the incision itself is very small. It is a stab incision with a width of 5 mm to 7 mm. Drainage is then obtained through blunt dissection with a hemostat. A large incision will only increase the trauma to the tissues and possibly damage larger blood vessels and nerves. A rubber drain, to be removed in 24 to 48 hours, helps with residual pus drainage and seems to speed up swelling resolution.

❖   The extraction may be done at the same visit when a patient presents with an acute infection caused by a tooth that you see will not require osteotomy in order to be removed. If there is facial cellulitis, prescribe antibiotics along with performing the extraction and incision and drainage. Consider having the patient start the antibiotics with a double dose, such as 1000 mg of amoxicillin instead of 500 mg, one hour

5 Kuriyama T1, Absi EG, Williams DW, Lewis MA. An outcome audit of the treatment of acute dentoalveolar infection: impact of penicillin resistance. *Br Dent J*. 2005 Jun 25; 198(12):759-63; Hargraves K, Cohen S. *Cohen's Pathways of the Pulp*. Tenth Edition. Elsevier Publishing; 2011, p. 42.

before the extraction is done, thereafter taking the usual antibiotic dose (if it is amoxicillin, 500 mg every 8 hours). Studies show that, in the presence of an acute infection, there is less systemic involvement if the tooth is extracted (along with performing incision and drainage and prescribing antibiotics) than if it is left in place and the only treatment provided is antibiotic therapy along with incision and drainage.[6]

Instruments

❖ **2 hourigan modified woodson periosteal elevator** (Hu-Friedy, Chicago, IL). Great for syndesmotomy, for extraction of root tips and as an elevator for remaining roots.

❖ **301 elevator with a serrated tip.** Very useful for removal of remaining roots and third molars with conical roots

❖ **150 forceps and 151 forceps.** Most extractions can be done using one of these two forceps.

❖ **Cowhorn forceps.** For mandibular 1st and 2nd molars with non-retentive roots.

❖ **New 557 carbide long shank bur.** For sectioning roots and performing osteotomy.

❖ **New 332 carbide bur.** For sectioning the crown off. It cuts enamel and dentin quickly when new.

❖ **Dental Surgical Headlight.** Greatly improves visibility of root tips in upper posterior areas.

❖ **Impact Air 45 Highspeed Handpiece** (Palisades Dental, Englewood, NJ). For osteotomy and root sectioning during surgical extraction. Air is exhausted through the back of the handpiece preventing air embolism from occurring.

---

6 Igoumenakis D, Giannakopoulos N, Parara E, Mourouzis C, Rallis G. Effect of Causative Tooth Extraction on Clinical and Biological Parameters of Odontogenic Infection: A Prospective Clinical Trial. *J Oral Maxillofac Surg.* 2015 Jul; 73(7):1254-8; Johri A, Piecuch JF. Should teeth be extracted immediately in the presence of acute infection? *Oral Maxillofac Surg Clin North Am.* 2011 Nov; 23(4): 507-11.

❖ **Cawood-Minnesota Retractor** (Hu-Friedy, Chicago, IL). Used to hold mucoperiosteal flaps, cheeks, lips, and tongue away from the surgical area. It works much better than a mouth mirror for retracting soft tissues during an extraction.

❖ As a general rule, do not purchase cheap instruments. Usually, a more expensive instrument has better quality and will make your work easier and quicker, benefiting both the patient and you.

❖ For deciduous teeth, instead of forceps, use a very small rongeur (upper or lower, depending on the tooth). It grips deciduous teeth very well. Also, your hand will hide it completely so as to provoke less fear in the patient.

Pain and Anxiety Control

❖ Consider telling the patient before you start the extraction: "You are going to feel some pressure and you may hear some noises but if you feel any pain at all, please let me know. If it hurts, lift your hand and I will stop immediately. As soon as you lift your hand I will stop." By saying this to the patient, and acting accordingly, you give him a sense of control and you diminish his level of apprehension. If the patient signals to you, stop and administer more anesthesia.

❖ While doing an extraction, pay attention to the patient's facial expression and hands. If you see the patient wincing, closing his eyes tightly, tightening his grip on the arm rest, or other similar sign, stop what you are doing and ask him: "Is it hurting?" If the patient tells you that it is, administer more anesthesia before going on with the procedure. This also applies to any other treatment you are performing such as drilling a tooth or instrumenting a canal. No one likes to feel pain.

Prior to the Extraction

❖ Always have the patient sign a consent form prior to the extraction.

❖   IMPORTANT: Do not let the patient wait for a long time once it is decided that an extraction will be done. The less time you keep the patient waiting, the less time he is kept in fear and distress.

❖   Have the assistant dab Vaseline on the patient's lips. This will reduce his discomfort if his lips must be pulled and stretched.

❖   Do not let the patient see the extraction instruments. Keep them on a tray placed behind the patient and covered with a sterilized napkin. Even though patients normally do not say anything when they see the instruments, the sight of them will usually increase their fear and apprehension.

❖   Have the assistant set up the tray after the patient has been seated in the dental chair.

Performing the Extraction

❖   Separate the soft tissues from the tooth carefully and well. The less trauma to the soft tissue, the less post-operative discomfort the patient will have.

❖   When sectioning a tooth or performing osteotomy, avoid using a conventional high-speed handpiece. The air jet that it releases into the surgical field may cause an air embolism.[7] There are surgical handpieces, such as Impact Air mentioned earlier, which do not spray air into the surgical field.

❖   Often, 1st molars have roots that spread out wider than the diameter of the tooth and the surrounding bone structure at the cervical area. When this is the case, for the tooth to come out of the socket, some fracture must happen. Usually, it is the crown that fractures off or one of the roots but, occasionally, it can be the alveolar bone that fractures. To avoid this possibility, it is best to section the tooth and remove the roots separately. This greatly reduces the risk of injury to bone and soft tissue. By sectioning the tooth and removing the roots separately you

---

7 Romeo, Umberto et al. Subcutaneous emphysema during third molar surgery: a case report. *Braz. Dent. J.* [online]. 2011, vol.22, n.1 pp.83-86.

do not have to pull something big through a small hole. Instead, you pull something small—the single root, through a bigger diameter hole—the alveolar socket at the cervical area. Also, you reduce the amount of force necessary to remove the tooth. Less force, less chances of bone fracture, less stress at the TMJ if it is a mandibular molar, less discomfort to the patient.

❖ As a rule, do not extract an unsectioned maxillary 1st molar unless there is moderate to advanced bone loss. The X-ray image of this tooth may give the false impression of bunched, conical roots but usually the palatal root is at an angle to the other roots. If you attempt to extract a maxillary 1st molar without separating the roots first, there is a possibility that a portion of the fragile alveolar buccal bone plate will fracture and come out with the tooth.

❖ Before applying pulling forces or, if it is a tooth that you plan to section, before sectioning, apply luxating forces to the tooth with the forceps for a minute or so. You can apply a buccal-lingual force and a rotational force (even in multirooted teeth, as long as the amplitude of the movement is very small—a few millimeters at the tip of the handle of the forceps). The purpose of the luxation movement is to rupture the periodontal ligament fibers and slightly widen the alveolar socket. The extraction, once this is done, will usually require less force than if the periodontal attachment is intact. And, if there is a root fracture during the extraction, the remaining root fragment will likely be loose in the socket and can be easily coaxed out as opposed to it being firmly attached to the socket walls by the periodontal ligament fibers when no luxating movement is done.

❖ Prior to sectioning a tooth, remove the coronal 3/4 of the crown. The reasons for doing this are: (1) with the coronal tooth structure out, you will have much better visibility as you section the roots within bone; (2) if the coronal tooth structure is not removed, due to the shape of the roots, its parts will get in the way and block each other as you try to wiggle a section out. Often the roots in mandibular molars are curved, similar to the shape of forceps handles, and converge at the crown. The maxillary roots are usually splayed out and converge at the crown. When the crown is removed, the roots have space to move into as they are separately extracted from the socket. The reason to leave a couple of millimeters of tooth above the gingiva is to have a surface that the elevator tip can engage, or for the forceps to grasp.

❖ When you section the coronal tooth structure horizontally to remove the crown, be careful not to touch the neighboring teeth with the bur. One way to be sure to avoid this is to drill a channel through the crown and leave 1 mm of tooth structure at the mesial and distal interproximal walls. You can then place a straight, flat elevator into the drilled channel and, with a twist of the wrist, pop the coronal tooth structure out without having gone too close to the neighboring teeth with the bur.

❖ For each tooth that you section, use a new set of burs. A sharp bur will greatly reduce the time required to complete this procedure.

❖ When examining the X-ray of a maxillary posterior tooth, make a mental note of the location of the maxillary sinus in relation to its roots. Often the roots are very close to the sinus and, occasionally, the antral cavity can extend in between the roots, especially between the 2nd premolar and 1st molar. If one is not careful, one may cause a perforation of the sinus floor as one sections the roots. To prevent this from occurring, use the bur with care, with clear vision provided by adequate suctioning, lighting, and magnification, while keeping in mind the anatomy seen on the X-ray.

❖ Sometimes, even after luxating a molar, sectioning its crown off and separating its roots, it can still be difficult to obtain root movement. When this is the case, a 3 mm depth osteotomy with a 557 bur along the mesio-buccal line angle of the mesial-buccal root if it is a maxillary molar, or the mesial root if it is a mandibular molar, will permit you to insert a 301 elevator deeper against the root. This will provide leverage. Once the tip of the 301 elevator is between the mesial wall of the socket and the root, a gentle rotation of the instrument along its long axis, will usually obtain root movement.

❖ Pay attention to the shape of the roots when looking at an X-ray. For example: in a mandibular 1st molar (which has already been sectioned) in which the mesial root curves toward the distal, you will know to use an elevator to remove this root, instead of a forceps, and to apply force in a distal direction.

❖   In premolars try to place the forceps as far apically (always over tooth structure) as it will go. Remember to make a luxation movement for about 1 minute prior to applying pulling forces to the tooth.

❖   When extracting a mandibular tooth always use a bite block as this greatly reduces the pressure transmitted to the patient's TMJ. Also, never use strong force because it may cause bone fracture and/or damage to the TMJ. If you have used gentle force and placed a bite block, make sure to enter it in the chart: "Placed bite block, used gentle force."

❖   When it is an incisor that will be extracted due to advanced bone loss, you can, prior to the extraction, bond the coronal portion of the tooth to the adjacent teeth. Then, section the tooth at the level of the gingiva and extract the root. After removing the root, from the lingual surface, grind into the pulp chamber and canal space to remove any pulpal debris. If the pulp is left in place, the crown will darken and become unaesthetic. Fill the pulp chamber and canal space with composite and, with a multifluted finishing bur, adjust the gingival portion of the crown-pontic. Before starting this procedure explain to the patient that this is a temporary option for tooth replacement.

❖   Avoid reflecting a flap, if possible, as this can increase post-operative discomfort. If a root fractures during an extraction, the first step is to be able to see it well. Magnification, adequate lighting, and adequate suction to remove blood from the socket will allow you to see the root, even if it is with indirect vision, that is, looking at its reflection in a mouth mirror. Once you see the root clearly, you can try to tease it out with a root tip pick or a bent explorer tip. If the tooth was well luxated prior to pulling it with the forceps, the root tip may be loose. If, however, it is not coming out, you can attempt to section it, or you can do an osteotomy around one of its surfaces using a 557 long shank bur. This will usually loosen the root and will provide you with a point of purchase from which to apply lateral pressure to it. When doing the osteotomy, it is very important to keep in mind the surrounding anatomy. Always stay away from the lingual alveolar wall in mandibular teeth and, on any tooth, go only about 3 mm deep with the bur before attempting again to use an elevator. Place the instrument in the groove you just created and apply lateral pressure. In most cases this is sufficient to remove the root avoiding the need for a flap reflection and extensive osteotomy. The key in this procedure is to have a clear view of the root, <u>with magnification</u>.

When the remaining root is in an upper posterior area, it can be difficult to obtain adequate illumination of the socket. In this case, a dental surgical headlight will greatly increase visibility.

After the Extraction

❖   After the extraction, run a finger over the gingiva at the alveolar border of the tooth socket, feeling for sharp bony edges. If you detect a sharp edge through the gingiva, remove it with a bone file or rongeur. If the sharp bony edge is not removed, it may eventually perforate the gingiva causing pain and discomfort to the patient.

❖   Use a resorbable suture if suture is needed. When, for some reason, the patient cannot return in one week to your office for a follow-up visit, the suture will come off by itself.

❖   After an extraction, give the post-operative instructions clearly. Make sure the patient understands what he is being told. Write your cell number in the post op instruction sheet. Give him, along with the post-op instruction sheet, sterilized gauze in a pouch and a plastic bag with ice so that he can already start applying cold to his face on the way home. The better the patient understands your instructions and follows them, the less chance there is of a dry socket developing.

❖   Prescribe pain medication if you sense that the patient will be in pain, such as when an incision and osteotomy are required.

❖   Call the patient at night, on the day of the extraction, to ask how he is doing.

❖   When the patient returns a few days after an extraction with the complaint that he feels pain whenever he touches a certain area, or that he feels something sharp that hurts whenever he touches it, it is likely a sharp edge of the alveolar socket that has punched through the gingiva/mucosa (bone spicule). If this is the case, it will usually look like an ulceration with a hard white center and the patient will feel pain when you touch it. The treatment is: 1. numb the area; 2. reflect flap if necessary; 3. remove sharp bony edge with bone file; 4. feel with your finger, over gingiva/mucosa, to make sure there are no sharp edges left; 5. suture if flap was reflected.

Chapter 11

IMPLANTS

Biology of Osseointegration

Osseointegration is the direct functional and structural connection between bone and the surface of a load bearing implant.

Contact Osteogenesis: When bone progenitor cells migrate to the implant surface and form bone directly in contact with the implant.

Distance Osteogenesis: When bone forms at the border of the osteotomy and progresses toward the implant.

The literature suggests that the main factor affecting the formation of a fibrous encapsulation around implants is micromotion of the implant. The threshold of micromotion that still allows for osseointegration is between 50 and 150 microns.[1] Stability of the implant, that is, lack of micromotion over 150 microns, therefore, seems to be what promotes osseointegration.

Stability of the implant is achieved in 2 steps:

1) Primary stability is obtained by the implant being slightly larger than the drilled hole and occurs immediately at placement.

2) Secondary stability occurs by the gradual formation of bone directly in contact with the implant surface and is achieved in two or more months.

Implant Shape, Surface, and Size

❖ There is a higher success rate for implants with microrough surface—2 to 3 microns rugosity—than implants with machined

---

1 Szmukler-Moncler, Salama H, Reingewirtz Y, Dubruille JH. Timing of loading and effect of micromotion on bone-dental implant interface: review of experimental literature. *J Biomed Mater Res.* 1998 Summer; 43(2):192-203.

surface—less than 0.5 microns rugosity.[2] Microrough surfaces are characterized by both contact and distance osteogenesis, whereas in machined surfaces only distance osteogenesis occurs.

❖ Several studies have shown that implants as short as 6 mm in length can be highly successful in both the maxilla and mandible.[3]

❖ Literature reviews show that the implant/crown ratio can be up to 1/2.5 and it will still have a normal success rate. This occurs even in 6 mm length implants.[4]

Types of Implants

❖ Endosseous implant is a two-piece implant. It consists in the endosseous part and the transmucosal part (abutment) that goes on top of it. The endosseous implant is normally placed at the level of the bone and the abutment is screwed into place after the surgery.

❖ Transmucosal implant is a one-piece implant. It is composed of both the endosseous and transmucosal portions. The transmucosal implant is placed so that its top is one or more millimeters above the bone and the gingiva is sutured around it.

❖ Narrow implants are preferred in the following situations:

1) Small distance between adjacent roots, such as in the mandibular anterior region.

2 Lambert FE1, Weber HP, Susarla SM, Belser UC, Gallucci GO. Descriptive analysis of implant and prosthodontic survival rates with fixed implant-supported rehabilitations in the edentulous maxilla. *J Periodontol.* 2009 Aug; 80(8):1220-30.
3 Anitua E1, Alkhraisat MH2. 15-year follow-up of short dental implants placed in the partially edentulous patient: Mandible Vs maxilla. *Ann Anat.* 2019 Mar; 222: 88-93. Esfahrood ZR1, Ahmadi L2, Karami E2, Asghari S3. Short dental implants in the posterior maxilla: a review of the literature. *J Korean Assoc Oral Maxillofac Surg.* 2017 Apr; 43(2): 70-76. Epub 2017 Apr 25. Telleman G et al. A systematic review of the prognosis of short (<10 mm) dental implants placed in the partially edentulous patient. J *Clin Periodontol.* 2011 Jul; 38(7): 667-76 Epub 2011 May 12.
4 Henny J. A. Meijer,corresponding author 1 , 2 Carina Boven, 1 Konstantina Delli, 1 and Gerry M. Raghoebar 1. Is there an effect of crown-to-implant ratio on implant treatment outcomes? A systematic review. *Clin Oral Implants Res.* 2018 Oct; 29(Suppl Suppl 18): 243–252.

2) Thin ridge, such as is often the case also in the mandibular anterior region.

❖ Tapered implants

Have denser thread distribution, threads that are closer to the apex. They provide improved primary stability and are more congruent to the bed in an extraction socket. They are used in:

1) Extraction sockets.

2) Type 4 bone.

❖ Morse Taper implant

Contains an internal cone shaped implant/abutment connection.[5] Some of its advantages over other implants are:

1) A marked decrease in the microgap size within the abutment-implant joint, thus reducing biofilm accumulation.

2) Reduced resorption of crestal bone. This is attributed to the fact that this design incorporates a platform switch (explained below).

3) Morse taper implant-abutment design eliminates the need for additional screw retained connections associated with other implant-abutment designs.

4) The smaller abutment diameter in proportion to the implant diameter naturally provides for increased thickness of the connective soft tissue around the abutment.

❖ Platform Switch

Platform switch consists in using an abutment that has a smaller diameter than the collar of the implant. For example, an implant with a 4.8 mm collar diameter is restored with a 3.8 mm diameter abutment

5 Macedo JP, Pereira J, Vahey BR, et al. Morse taper dental implants and platform switching: The new paradigm in oral implantology. *Eur J Dent*. 2016;10(1):148–154.

leaving a 0.5 mm wide platform at the collar. In an implant where the implant/abutment junction is straight, that is, without a collar, once the abutment is placed, the bone will usually recede 1.5 to 2 mm from the implant-abutment junction. However, when a platform switch is used, the average vertical bone loss at the implant collar has been shown to be 0.75 mm.[6]

Types of Healing Protocols

❖   Endosseous implant with submerged healing is when the implant is covered by soft tissues during the healing phase. It is preferred:

1) When a soft tissue born temporary will be used. Submerged healing prevents that the temporary prosthesis transfer forces to the implant causing it to move and not osseointegrate.

2) When soft tissue intervention is planned for a later date.

3) In the esthetic zone because it allows for more prosthetic flexibility and more possibilities for soft tissue management.

❖   Transmucosal healing is when the soft tissues are sutured around the implant so that it is exposed to the oral environment.

1) Preferred in straightforward procedures such as in some posterior cases.

2) Simplifies prosthetic protocol.

Your First Implant

❖   Select a case with minimal complexity. Look for a healthy patient with good oral hygiene and realistic expectations. Replacement of a

6 Vela-Nebot X1, Rodríguez-Ciurana X, Rodado-Alonso C, Segalà-Torres. Benefits of an implant platform modification technique to reduce crestal bone resorption. *M Implant Dent*. 2006 Sep; 15(3): 313-20.

mandibular second premolar or first molar are usually the simplest cases.

❖   Start by determining the shape and location of the crown with which the implant will be restored. Know in detail the restorative phase of this treatment.

❖   Know in detail the anatomy of the field you will operate. Obtain a CT scan of the area to be operated. The panoramic X-ray alone does not provide sufficient anatomical information for a safe implant surgery to be undertaken.

❖   Ensure your patient is well informed and that he knows the risk factors.

❖   Rehearse well every procedure so that you will go into the surgery assured of yourself.

Risk Assessment

Serious risk factors

1) Bacterial plaque: If the patient cannot control plaque accumulation, it is best not to place the implant.

2) Active periodontal disease: It must be treated before an implant can be placed.

3) Radiation therapy of the jaws: This can be qualified as a prohibitive condition such as is active periodontal disease or noncompliance on the part of the patient.

Modifying factors

The following factors do not preclude implant placement but may adversely affect its success rate.

1) Diabetes: Compromised wound healing, greater susceptibility to periodontal disease and inflammation.

2) Smoking: Studies show a higher failure rate for smokers than for non-smokers. There is more inflammation and bone loss around implants in

smokers than in non-smokers.[7] Explain this to the patient and it may serve as a stimulus for him to quit smoking.

3) Anti-resorption medication: Consider referring to an oral surgeon. Intravenous intake of bisphosphonates monthly for cancer increases greatly the chances of osteonecrosis.

Predisposing factor

1) History of periodontitis. This factor also does not preclude implant placement. It means, however, that it must be emphasized to the patient that he will have to come in for six-month recall appointments for the remainder of his life. The fact that the patient has a history of periodontitis indicates he has susceptibility to this condition and that it may occur again.

Phases of Treatment

1) Initial exam, diagnosis: The panoramic X-ray does not allow one to determine bone width and quality. This must be determined with a CT scan. Use cone beam CT whenever possible.

2) Treatment planning: Do diagnostic wax up as part of this process. Determine which teeth have a good prognosis, which teeth have a doubtful prognosis, and which should be extracted.

3) Systemic phase: Make sure the patient is healthy, with illnesses such as high blood pressure and diabetes under control. Refer to a physician if there is any systemic condition that is untreated.

4) Hygiene phase: Includes restorative treatment. The patient must have optimal hygiene and be free of any gingival or periodontal inflammation or caries before the implants can be placed.

---

7 Bruno Ramos B, Albrektssona T, Wennerberga. Smoking and dental implants: A systematic review and meta-analysis. *Journal of Dentistry*. 2015 May; 43(5): 487-498.

5) Surgical phase: Consists in implant placement. Use a surgical stent where possible. Know well the anatomy of the area where surgery will be performed.

6) Prosthetic phase: Temporaries, when used, must be well made and atraumatic. The temporary assists in tissue conditioning. If it is rough, for example, plaque will accumulate and cause inflammation.

7) Maintenance phase: Regular maintenance hygiene appointments not only serve as a therapeutic measure but also as a motivational factor to the patient.

Some Points to Keep in Mind While Treatment Planning

❖   Do not assume the radiologist is correct in his interpretation of the X-rays. Evaluate them for yourself, carefully, as the responsibility for all that occurs during treatment is yours and not his.

❖   Ideally, there should be at least 1 mm of bone surrounding the implant.

❖   In adjacent implants, when the distance between them is more than 3 mm, the crestal bone loss between them has been shown to be 0.45 mm. Whereas when it is equal to or less than 3 mm, the bone loss has been shown to be 1.04 mm. Therefore, it is better to keep at least more than 3 mm space between implants.[8]

❖   Implant placement must be restorative driven, that is, you must place the implant in a position that will favor its restoration. Therefore, begin the treatment by determining what the final restoration will be and what will be its shape. Place the implants according to this planned prosthesis.

❖   After determining what the final prosthesis will be, have the lab do a diagnostic wax-up. This will help the patient visualize what the final restoration will look like and will serve as a guide for the fabrication of the surgical stent that will guide the implant placement.

---

8 Tarnow, DP1 et al. The effect of inter-implant distance on the height of inter-implant bone crest. *J Periodontology*. 2000 Apr; 71(4): 546-9.

❖   FPDs that are supported by both implants and teeth have a higher failure rate than do FPDs that are solely supported either by teeth or implants. One of the major complications that can happen with implant/teeth supported FPDs is intrusion of the abutment tooth. Therefore, it is better to avoid this type of treatment.[9]

❖   Full arch reconstruction in the mandible should ideally be separated into three separate bridges because of the bending of the mandible in maximum opening. This helps to prevent complications with the prosthesis.

❖   It is critical to make the first 1 to 2 millimeters of the subgingival part of the implant, that is, the gingival sulcus, accessible for oral hygiene. If not, plaque will accumulate in the area leading to inflammation and possible bone loss.

❖   A study demonstrated that patients who have a history of chronic periodontitis, but no active periodontitis, have an equal prognosis for implants as do healthy patients. That is, an equal chance of success. However, the same study shows that patients with active periodontitis have more bone loss and inflammation around implants than do healthy patients.[10]

❖   In cases where there is not enough bone to surround the implant in its entirety but there is enough to obtain primary stability, one can do implant placement and perform guided tissue regeneration simultaneously.

❖   At the treatment planning phase, mentally divide the implant into three segments – apical, middle and cervical. If one of the three segments is completely surrounded by bone, there is a good chance you will obtain primary stability and will be able to simultaneously place the implant and do guided bone regeneration.

❖   It is recommended to wait 6 to 8 weeks after an extraction before placing an implant. This allows for soft tissue coverage of the extraction socket and consequent primary closure of the implant surgical site. However, it is better not to wait six months for implant placement.

9 Albrektsson T1, Donos N. Implant survival and complications. The Third EAO consensus conference 2012. *Clin Oral Implants Res.* 2012 Oct; 23 Suppl 6: 63-5.
10 Cho-Yan Lee J1, Mattheos N, Nixon KC, Ivanovski S. Residual periodontal pockets are a risk indicator for peri-implantitis in patients treated for periodontitis. *Clin Oral Implants Res.* 2012 Mar; 23(3): 325-33. Epub 2011 Aug 5.

Studies show that six months after an extraction there is on average 3.8 mm horizontal resorption of alveolar ridge and 1.3 mm of vertical resorption of the ridge.[11]

❖ In an immediate placement in the anterior maxilla, place the implant preferably 2 mm towards the palate and 1 mm into the socket to allow for the bone resorption that will occur post extraction.

Cone Beam CT in Anterior Teeth

❖ Have the cone beam CT taken with the patient's lips and cheek being retracted. This is done using a lips and cheek retractor and it allows for a better visualization of the gingiva.

❖ Have the patient wear a splint with a radiopaque tooth at the site being restored. This allows you to determine the exact location for implant placement.

❖ Look for the incisive canal in the radiographic image.

Surgical Principles

1 – Be minimally invasive. The less invasive one is, the less trauma to the tissues.

2 – Be quick. The longer a surgery takes, the more complications can occur. Quickness is accomplished not so much by moving quickly but by knowing well each step of the surgery, having a competent assistant who knows ahead of time what you will need, and by streamlining the procedure, that is, by setting up a tray with the instruments you will need in the order they will be used.

3 – Have a proper suturing technique. Use 5.0 or 6.0 suture in order to reduce tension on the blood clot. The thin strand will snap before too much tension can be placed on the tissues.

---

11 Tan WL1, Wong TL, Wong MC, Lang NP. A systematic review of post-extractional alveolar hard and soft tissue dimensional changes in humans. *Clin Oral Implants Res.* 2012 Feb; 23 Suppl 5: 1-21.

Some useful instruments to have available during implant surgery:

- Universal periodontal scaler to remove granulation tissue.

- Bone curette for removing granulation tissue from inside a socket.

- Large intraoral mirror to help to determine if there is proper parallelism between implants.

- Head illumination in order to improve visibility.

Surgical Procedure

❖ Avoid vertical releasing incisions when placing a single implant that does not need a bone graft. Releasing incisions increase post-op discomfort and prolong the healing phase.

❖ Prepare a 2 to 3 mm deep entry site with a round drill.

❖ Use plenty of irrigation during osteotomy to avoid overheating the bone, compromising osseointegration. Studies show that when bone is heated above 47 C, osteocyte death occurs.[12]

❖ Drill solely with an up and down movement. Lateral, wobbly movements while drilling will create an inadequate implant placement site hampering osseointegration.

❖ Do not drill full length with the twist drill (the first sight drill). Drill part of the way and then check alignment. If the alignment is not good, it can still be changed at this point.

❖ In poor quality bone, make the diameter of the implant socket smaller than the diameter of the implant itself to give it stability.

❖ The maximum force used to seat an implant must not exceed 60 N. When the force necessary to screw in the implant is over 60 N, it may either damage the implant or cause excessive compression on the bone, affecting osseointegration. If the implant is not penetrating into the socket with the recommended force, the osteotomy site must be enlarged slightly with additional screw tapping. This can be

12 Dolan EB, Haugh MG, Voisin MC, Tallon D, McNamara LM. Thermally induced osteocyte damage initiates a remodelling signaling cascade. *PLoS One*. 2015;10(3): e0119652. Published 2015 Mar 18.

accomplished also by using the implant itself as a screw tap. With the manual torque wrench, unscrew the implant a few turns, without removing it completely from the osteotomy site. Then screw it again. Stop when the force required reaches 50 N, unscrew the implant a few turns, screw it again and so forth until the implant is fully seated in the implant bed.

❖ Take a post-op X-ray immediately after implant placement to ensure that the teeth have not been damaged and that important anatomical structures are intact.

Sinus Lift

❖ After detaching the sinus membrane (Schneiderian membrane) have the patient gently inhale while you watch the membrane. If it moves into the sinus, it is a sign that there is no perforation. One in every five sinus elevation procedures results in a sinus perforation.[13] A tip to avoid perforation of the sinus membrane: concentrate on gently tracing the sinus bony floor and walls with your instrument. This will automatically lift the membrane.

❖ A sinus membrane perforation can be closed with resorbable suture or by covering it with a collagenous membrane. If left open, a perforation of the sinus membrane increases the risk of sinusitis by impairment of functional homeostasis and by dispersion of the graft material into the antral cavity, making it more prone to infection.[14]

❖ About 70 % of atrophy of the posterior area of the maxilla that occurs after an extraction is resorption of the alveolar ridge; thirty percent is expansion of the sinus.[15]

13 Pjetursson BE1, Tan WC, Zwahlen M, Lang NP. A systematic review of the success of sinus floor elevation and survival of implants inserted in combination with sinus floor elevation. *J Clin Periodontol*. 2008 Sep; 35(8 Suppl): 216-40.
14 Deborah Meleo, DDS, PhD,1 Francesca Mangione, DDS,1 Sergio Corbi, MD, DDS,2 and Luciano Pacifici, MD, DDS1. Management of the Schneiderian membrane perforation during the maxillary sinus elevation procedure: a case report. *Ann Stomatol (Roma)*. 2012 Jan-Mar; 3(1): 24–30.
15 Cavalcanti, Marilia et al. Maxillary sinus floor pneumatization and alveolar ridge resorption after tooth loss: a cross-sectional study. *Brazilian Oral Research*. 2018; vol 32

❖   Guidelines for choosing between the osteotome technique or the lateral window technique:

-   8 mm of bone should be enough for the placement of an implant without sinus elevation.

-   6 to 7 mm of bone and a flat sinus floor are indicated for the osteotome technique.

-   4 to 5 mm of bone and a flat sinus floor are indicated for osteotome with grafting material.

-   2 to 4 mm of bone, or an oblique sinus floor, should be treated with a lateral window approach. Immediate implant placement is done if primary stability can be obtained.

-   1 to 2 mm of bone should be treated with a lateral window sinus lift followed by a waiting period of 6 to 9 months for implant placement.

Suturing

❖   The more tension there is on a suture, the more tension there will be on the underlying clot. The greater the tension on the clot, the greater the damage to the clot and the longer it will take for healing to occur. A clot under tension resorbs and revascularizes slower than one that is not under tension.

❖   During the first 24 hours, trauma from the suture is mechanical. From then on, it is bacterial. To reduce bacterial proliferation there are suture materials coated with triclosan.

❖   A way to prevent excessive tension on the tissues is to use thin sutures such as 5.0 or 6.0. They will usually break before tissue breaks, preventing excessive pressure from being applied to the tissues and blood clot. When a thin suture material is used, the tightness of the suture is determined visually and not with tactile sensation.

❖   To suture a perforated Schneiderian membrane, use a dull, round tipped needle and resorbable suture. A sharp needle will cause further tear to the membrane.

❖   The most precise human movement is the circular movement of the hand from the 2 o'clock position to the 7 o'clock position. Therefore, a pen grasp needle holder allows for more precise suturing than a scissor grasp needle holder.

❖   When suturing, pull the suture filament slowly through the tissue to avoid the sawing effect that occurs if it is pulled quickly.

❖   Monofilament sutures allow for less bacterial adherence than do polyfilament sutures. Sutures where the filament is glued to a hole drilled in the back end of the needle produce less tissue trauma than do sutures where the filament is clamped to the needle.

Post-Operative Period

❖   Prior to dismissing the patient after a surgical procedure, warn him of what to expect during the first few days following surgery. Explain that there may be pain, swelling, bleeding, and bruising and show him how to minimize these through proper postoperative care.

❖   The post-operatory period after a simple implant procedure is similar to that of a simple extraction. When bone augmentation is also performed, however, there is more swelling and pain than in a simple implant procedure. Swelling is normally greatest in the second day post-surgery.

❖   A small lingual perforation of the mandible during implant placement can cause damage to a salivary gland or a blood vessel. This often goes unnoticed and will result in a gradual seepage of fluids into the sublingual area, causing the tongue to be lifted obstructing the airway – a life threatening situation. A way to prevent a lingual perforation from occurring is to know well the anatomy of the patient through a careful study of his cone beam tomography images. Swelling of the floor of the mouth, however, can occur even when there is no bony plate perforation, therefore, when giving the post-op instructions after implant placement in the mandible, ask the patient to call you immediately if he feels swelling occurring in the floor of the mouth.[16]

16 Peñarrocha-Diago M, et al José Carlos Balaguer-Martí, David Peñarrocha-Oltra, José Bagán, Miguel Peñar[show]. Floor of the mouth hemorrhage subsequent to dental

Possible Complications of Implant Surgery

1) Hemorrhage

2) Nerve injury

3) Injury to adjacent teeth

4) Implant fracture or damage

Prosthetic Procedures

❖ Several studies show that 4 to 6 implants suffice to support a full-arch restoration, whether in the maxilla or in the mandible. The minimum number of implants for a full-arch implant supported restoration is 4 implants.[17]

❖ Patients with bruxism have significantly more prosthetic complications than patients without. Cantilever extensions are also associated with more failures than implant supported FPDs without a cantilever.[18]

❖ In a study by Nedir et al, overdentures were shown to have more complications than fixed restorations. The complications were recurrent and usually simple to adjust. Bar-retained overdentures had significantly less complications than ball-retained overdentures.[19]

❖ When choosing between screw-retained and cemented restorations, screw-retained restorations should be the first choice because of retrievability and because in cement retained restorations,

implant placement in the anterior mandible. *Clinical, Cosmetic and Investigational Dentistry.* August 2019, vol 11.

17 Mericske-Stern R, Worni A. Optimal number of oral implants for fixed reconstructions: a review of the literature. *Eur J Oral Implantol.* 2014 Summer;7 Suppl 2: S133-53.

18 Brägger U1, Aeschlimann S, Bürgin W, Hämmerle CH, Lang NP. Biological and technical complications and failures with fixed partial dentures (FPD) on implants and teeth after four to five years of function. *Clin Oral Implants Res.* 2001 Feb; 12(1): 26-34.

19 Nedir R1, Bischof M, Szmukler-Moncler S, Belser UC, Samson J. Prosthetic complications with dental implants: from an up-to-8-year experience in private practice. *Int J Oral Maxillofac Implants.* 2006 Nov-Dec; 21(6): 919-28.

excess cement can penetrate the periimplant space causing inflammation and possible bone destruction.

❖   A general rule for determining the length of a cantilever in an implant restoration: multiply the distance between the middle of the most anterior implant and the distal part of the most posterior implant by 1.5. The resulting number is an estimate of the permissible distance for the cantilever length.[20]

❖   Immediate loading of an implant, that is, to restore it at the time of placement, is done only if there is primary stability. Some factors that enhance primary stability of an implant: aggressive, deep threads; diameter of the prepared implant site slightly smaller than the implant itself; angled, long implants.

❖   If a surgical stent is used for the implant placement surgery, the lab that fabricated the stent can also fabricate a temporary restoration which can then be placed postoperatively if immediate loading is planned.

❖   In order to immediately load an implant, ideally micromovement should be less than 50 microns. If it is more, connective tissue will likely form at implant interface.

❖   The periodontal ligament sensory apparatus lets the patient subconsciously know the direction and intensity of the forces being applied to the teeth. The masticatory muscles then adjust the position of the mandible so that the person automatically chews in a way in which the forces are applied to the long axis of the teeth. Dental implants, however, lack the periodontal ligament sensory apparatus, and consequently do not provide feedback regarding direction and intensity of the forces. Therefore, when the patient who has dental implants chews, he may inadvertently direct the chewing forces in a non-axial path. These forces are damaging to the restoration. To diminish their damaging effects, avoid implant restorations with deep cuspal inclinations and large occlusal tables.[21]

---

20 http://webstore.lexi.com/sample-pages/pdf/modi-2.pdf

21 Trulsson M. Sensory and motor function of teeth and dental implants: a basis for osseoperception. *Clin Exp Pharmacol Physiol.* 2005 Jan-Feb; 32(1-2): 119-22.

Immediate loading – When the implant is restored up to 1 week after implant placement surgery.

Early loading – When the implant is restored from 1 week up to 2 months after implant placement surgery.

Conventional loading – Restoration more than 2 months after implant placement surgery.

Mandibular Overdenture

❖ The full denture must be well constructed and achieve retention, stability, and support from the underlying tissues. The implant retainers serve only to enhance retention.
❖ The implant fixtures should be as parallel as possible and placed at the same height. If the implants are not parallel, component problems are more likely to happen later.
❖ When treatment planning, explain to the patient that, with time, the denture-bearing area will resorb, and the denture will need a reline.

Temporary Crown

❖ Provisionals help to condition the soft tissue that surrounds the implant.
❖ From a soft tissue conditioning perspective, ideally a temporary crown should be placed at the time of implant placement. But if there is no primary stability of the implant, then it is better to delay the placement of a temporary. Otherwise, micromovement caused by function will result in fibrous encapsulation.
❖ When doing soft tissue remodeling through the provisional crown, the provisional should be used for approximately three months prior to final restoration fabrication.
❖ The provisional should have no interfering occlusal contacts as this may affect osseointegration.
❖ In a submerged anterior implant, a fixed, well-polished temporary that is attached to the adjacent teeth, such as a Maryland Bridge, can be

used. This allows the healing gingival tissues that cover the implant to take a natural shape and form interdental papillae as they adapt around the temporary pontic.

Impression Taking

❖   When taking an impression of the implant, after removing the healing abutment make sure there is no soft tissue growth over the implant. Examine the entire circumference of the implant with a mirror. Soft tissue will prevent the proper seating of the definitive abutment.

❖   There cannot be contact between an impression coping and an adjacent tooth. If there is, it may prevent the coping from seating properly into the fixture. After seating the impression coping, use a metal matrix or floss to check if there is space between the tooth and the coping. If the metal matrix or floss does not go through easily, grind the coping until you are sure there is no contact.

❖   After seating the impression coping and having made any necessary adjustments to it, take an X-ray to make sure it is seated properly. If the implant threads appear clearly, it is a sign that there is parallelism of the X-ray with the implant, and the image will show whether the impression coping is properly seated.

Ceramic Complications

❖   Implant-supported ceramic restorations have a much higher failure rate than tooth-supported restorations because implants do not have the shock absorbing features of the periodontal ligament.

❖   When ceramic occludes against ceramic there is a higher incidence of chipping than when ceramic occludes with acrylic or against a natural tooth. The chipping usually occurs in the maxilla due to the force direction being diagonal to the long axis of the implant. A strategy to reduce porcelain chipping when implant restoration occludes with implant restoration is to restore one with acrylic and the other with porcelain.

❖ In an implant supported FPD, if there is any tension in the metal framework once it is seated on the abutments, it will be transferred to the porcelain resulting in eventual porcelain fracture. To avoid this, make sure every step of the impression process is free of error and check that the framework fits passively.

❖ As mentioned previously, the lack of mechanoceptors in an implant causes a greater amount of angular chewing forces to be directed at the restoration. Therefore, the occlusal table should be completely free of interferences, and as flat as possible, that is, without sharp cuspal inclinations.

❖ All porcelain should be supported by metal coping. If it is not, it will likely eventually fracture. Also, the porcelain should be of equal thickness. This allows for a better distribution of the forces diminishing the chances of porcelain fracture. Look at the restoration try-in X-ray to determine if the crown has these two features. If it does not, consider having the lab fabricate a new restoration. It may be an inconvenience at that moment, but it will prevent the greater inconvenience of a failed restoration.

When Treatment Is Finished?

1) Establish baseline records.

2) Establish a risk profile. Factors that increase risk: bruxism, history of periodontitis, smoking, diabetes, oral hygiene, previous implant complications.

3) Based on the above information, establish how often you will see the patient for the rest of his life.

The Three Things to Be Reviewed at Follow Up Visits

1) The patient: look for changes in the medical history or behavior, such as, if the patient has started smoking.

2) The implant.

3) The surrounding tissues: bleeding index, plaque index, calculus, inflammation, probing depth as compared to baseline probing depths, recession, bone loss.

Maintenance Phase

First step: Assess risk

Confirm whether the patient has a history of any of the following risk factors or has acquired it since the last visit: 1 - Poor oral hygiene; 2 – Diabetes; 3 - Periodontal disease; 4 - Smoking

Second step: Gently probe around implant

If there is bleeding, it is a sign of inflammation and most likely that oral hygiene needs to be improved. It could also be a sign of excess cement or an ill-fitting prosthesis with open spaces for bacterial colonization at the implant and/or prosthesis components. Unlike teeth, a probing depth of 4 or 5 mm around an implant does not necessarily mean there is inflammation since in implants there are no periodontal fibers closing off space between implant and soft tissue. Therefore, look for bleeding and compare your findings with the baseline findings.

Third step: Treat periimplantitis if it is present

1 – Modify the prosthesis if necessary, so that the patient will have better access for hygiene.

2 – Debride the implant with a rubber coated ultrasonic cleaner, prescribe a chlorhexidine mouth rinse. If this does not cure the periimplantitis, surgery is necessary.

3 – Surgical treatment (required in most cases) is done in order to access and decontaminate the implant surface.

The most effective way to address periimplantitis is to prevent it from occurring. A well-designed prosthesis, that allows the patient to have access to all surfaces of the implant for hygiene, and regular maintenance recalls, which not only help to keep the implants clean but serve also to motivate the patient, are important factors in preventing periimplantitis.[22]

<u>At the recall visit, when examining an X-ray of an implant and its restoration, look for:</u>

Biologically: Bone loss, apical periimplantitis.

Implant and prosthesis: Cracks, fractures, excess cement, loose screw, gaps.

Thread sharpness: If threads on both sides of the implants are sharp there is proper angulation between the X-ray cone and the implant. If the left side of the implant is sharp and the right side is blurry that means the cone is pointing down at the implant, that is, the X-ray comes from above. If the right side is sharp and the left is blurry, the X-ray comes from below.

The tilt of the sensor or film (not the X-ray cone), on the other hand, does not affect the sharpness of the image. It does affect its length, however.

General Points

What to do if you place and restore implants

1) Before placing the implant, ensure the patient has good oral hygiene.

2) Design implant prosthesis so as to allow access for oral hygiene.

3) Design the occlusion free of damaging interferences, while guiding occlusal forces apically.

4) Ensure tension-free (passive) fitness of the bridge framework.

---

22 Serino G1, Ström C. Peri-implantitis in partially edentulous patients: association with inadequate plaque control. *Clin Oral Implants Res.* 2009 Feb; 20(2): 169-74.

5) Follow all manufacturer's instructions and scientific guidelines and document every step.

6) Use an implant system you trust which is supported by good scientific evidence.

7) Avoid mixing components from different implant systems.

8) Document all information about the implant placed (size, system, type).

9) Give a plastic implant ID-card to your patients with information about the implant such as size, type, brand, date placed and a baseline radiograph. This is done so that if the patient moves or must see another dentist for any reason, the dentist will have access to this information.

Chapter 12

FIXED PARTIAL DENTURE

Prior to Starting

❖ Prior to starting an FPD treatment, explore with the patient all the options available to replace his missing tooth (teeth). Clearly explain the advantages and disadvantages of each option. Illustrate your points with lab cases that you may have waiting to be delivered or with lab cases that you have specifically for this purpose. Usually, an implant supported prosthesis is the best treatment available, with the best prognosis for the prosthesis itself and for the neighboring teeth. If your patient is concerned about the treatment cost, an example that you can give is that it is a much better investment than a new car. The implant treatment costs less and he will use it 24/7 (even while he is sleeping, it is a benefit by preventing extrusion of opposing teeth) for many years while the car is used only a few hours a day and usually does not last as long.

❖ If the patient's teeth are dark, offer bleaching to him prior to starting the treatment. Explain that the shade of the porcelain does not change with bleaching and that, if he wishes to have lighter teeth, bleaching should be done prior to FPD fabrication.

❖ Avoid cantilever FPDs since, with time, the porcelain tends to fracture and/or the FPD may come off. A possible candidate for a cantilever FPD would be a small person with weak masticatory muscles. The pontic should be as small in a mesial distal direction as aesthetics will permit to minimize the leverage for dislodging forces. Yet, even in such a patient, and with the conservative design described, an implant would still be a far better treatment option than a cantilever FPD.

❖ Check the occlusion and periodontal condition carefully prior to starting treatment. This is obvious but it does not hurt to mention it.

❖   The periodontal condition must be healthy for an FPD to be placed. Otherwise, abutments may become loose in a few years and the patient will lose the FPD along with his teeth. Also, if a patient has a history of periodontal disease, he must demonstrate good compliance with the periodontal maintenance appointments and adequate oral hygiene before an FPD is placed.

❖   Prior to preparing vital teeth for an FPD, carefully examine the X-ray image of the pulp chamber of each tooth. In posterior teeth, bitewing X-rays show well its dimensions. Try to determine if, to obtain a path of insertion, you will have to grind into pulp space. If you determine this may happen, it is better to include the RCT and post (if the RCT is on a molar, a core build up will usually suffice) in your treatment plan. If one fails to detect this possibility and finds out only after starting the tooth reduction that the crown preparation will go into the pulp chamber, it will create an uncomfortable situation with the patient. One must stop the procedure to tell him that, besides the two or more crown preparations, a RCT and core build up (with its additional cost and treatment time) will be necessary. Most patients will be displeased with the additional, unexpected cost and some may see this as a mistake on the dentist's part (or lack of foresight).

❖   Just as it occurs in single crown preparations, even if there is no pulp exposure, vital teeth may become necrotic or develop irreversible pulpitis after tooth reduction, in which case RCT will be necessary. Warn the patient of this possibility when first presenting him the treatment plan.

❖   When one is placing an FPD which includes one or more anterior teeth, it is advisable to use a laboratory-made temporary FPD instead of one fabricated chairside. The main reason for this is that the lab-made temporary FPD is usually much more aesthetic than one made in office. A couple of other reasons are: (1) you can request the lab- made temporary to be reinforced with metal, which makes it stronger than an all acrylic temporary FPD; (2) it saves chair time at the FPD preparation appointment because the temporary is almost ready (the abutments just need to be relined with acrylic) as opposed to starting it from scratch while the patient is in the chair.

FPD Preparation

❖   What applies to crowns applies also to FPDs.

❖   Make sure there is parallelism between the prepared abutments. If there is no parallelism, the FPD margins will be open. One way to check for this is with indirect vision, using a mirror long enough to show all prepared teeth at the same time. An intraoral photography mirror works well for this purpose. If you close one eye and can see all the margins when you look at the reflection in the mirror, there is parallelism between the prepared abutments and there is a path of insertion.

❖   Another way to check for parallelism is to make an alginate impression and pour it in fast set stone or pour it with a bite registration material (which sets quickly). Look at the model of the prepared teeth and check for parallelism and undercuts.

❖   Do not leave undercuts in any of the preparations.

❖   Always do a metal frame try-in when making an FPD. If there is an open margin, it will be detected prior to porcelain placement, saving the technician the effort of placing the porcelain, and also saving time for you and the patient because the problem will be detected earlier in the treatment sequence.

❖   In an FPD that includes one or more molars, do a bisque try-in instead of going directly to the glaze try-in. This is done to prevent sending the FPD too many times to the oven, which will make the porcelain brittle and liable to fracture. When extensive adjustment is done on the occlusal surfaces of several teeth, which is often the case in a posterior FPD, the FPD should be glazed afterwards to confer to it a glassy smooth surface. If the FPD has been glazed once already, the porcelain may become brittle due to it being placed in the oven at a very high temperature again. When the porcelain becomes brittle, a few years after cementing the prosthesis, or sooner, it may fracture.

❖   On an anterior FPD you may skip the bisque try-in and go directly to the finished case. That is, try-in the metal frame and then try-in the metal frame with the finished porcelain. The adjustments, if necessary, at the porcelain try-in, are usually small and on the lingual surface or incisal edge, allowing you to polish any ground areas with the proper rubber tips. If the lingual surface is in metal, it can be adjusted at the metal frame try-in so that at delivery often no adjustment is necessary.

The reason for trying in the FPD with the finished porcelain is because this will allow the patient to see the final aesthetics and make an informed decision whether he is pleased with it or not. If you do a bisque try-in, at the following appointment, with the porcelain glazed, the patient may decide he does not like the aesthetics. This makes the bisque try-in a wasted appointment, since the case will have to go back to lab again. It is wasted time for the patient and for you.

❖   It can be difficult to obtain closed margins on an FPD of six or more units (with the exception of a canine-to-canine FPD). If the patient needs such a treatment, consider referring him to a prosthodontist.

❖   Porcelain fused to metal (PFM) FPD 's seem, in clinical practice, to be more durable and have better margins than all-porcelain FPD's. If enough room is left for the porcelain when the abutments are prepared, and yellow gold is used for the metal core, the aesthetics of a PFM FPD is as good as that of an all-porcelain FPD. Also, less tooth reduction is required for a PFM FPD than for an all-porcelain FPD.

❖   When you are preparing the abutments, keep in mind whether the area you are grinding will be covered by porcelain and metal or just metal. The lingual surfaces of maxillary anterior teeth, for example, depending on the case, can be kept in metal. Less tooth reduction is required for metal only, leaving a stronger abutment and protecting the pulp, if the tooth is vital.

FPD Delivery

❖ Check the margins one more time prior to delivering an FPD, besides doing it at the metal frame try-in, and porcelain try-in for posterior FPD.

❖ If the abutments are vital, consider cementing the FPD with TempBond NE (Kerr, Orange, CA) or a similar temporary cement. In this way, if any of the abutments later need RCT, the FPD can be easily removed, and the RCT done, without a hole having to be drilled in the prosthesis. A good tap, with a crown and bridge remover, under the pontic will remove the FPD.

Post Op Instructions

❖ Post op instructions regarding shade: "The shade of the porcelain teeth will not change with time. Your teeth, in turn, may darken with time, in which case the prosthesis will no longer match their shade. If this happens, you can correct the difference with bleaching. Bleaching will lighten the shade of your teeth until it again resembles the shade of the porcelain."

❖ Show the patient how to clean under the pontic. There are hygiene items available for this such as dental floss threaders and interdental brushes. Give the patient a packet with the hygiene item of your preference. Interdental brushes seem to be easier to use than the floss threader.

❖ When the definitive FPD is cemented with temporary cement, it is important to let the patient know that this has been done and that the FPD can be removed. If, later, an abutment becomes symptomatic and the patient has moved away and cannot come to your office, he can tell his new dentist that the FPD is cemented with temporary cement. Thus, the dentist can remove it prior to RCT, instead of having to drill the endodontic access through the prosthesis.

Chapter 13

OCCLUSAL NIGHT GUARD

❖ Find an excellent lab to do this type of work for you. It may cost a little more, but the results are worth the additional expense. The ONG will require less adjustment than that of a laboratory that concentrates on quantity instead of quality. It will take less time to get it to fit and to adjust the occlusion.

❖ The impressions and models must be free of bubbles, defects and must not be distorted. The more faithful the models and bite registration are to the patient's oral structures (and the better the lab), the better the fit, that is, less adjustment necessary upon delivery.

❖ Make sure the ONG does not rock when it is in place. If it does, take a new impression, pour it immediately so that there is no time for the impression material to distort (teach the assistants to always pour alginate impressions immediately) and send the ONG back to the lab with the new model. The lab can first try to adjust the ONG to fit the new model. If this cannot be done, the lab can use the new model to fabricate a new ONG.

Another option when the ONG rocks, is to try to adjust it yourself with the help of a pressure indicating material, such as Fit Checker Pressure Indicator Paste (GC Corporation, Tokyo, Japan). This material shows where the ONG first touches the teeth. The downside of this approach is that it is time consuming and often does not work. After several adjustments one frequently finds that the ONG still rocks when it is in place. To avoid spending much time in an unsuccessful attempt to adjust the ONG, set a time limit for the procedure. For example, if after 5 minutes of adjustment the ONG still does not fit, stop, take an alginate impression, and send the case to the dental laboratory.

❖   Take your time adjusting the occlusion on an ONG to make it more comfortable to the patient and to prevent extrusion or shifting of teeth. All teeth must touch the ONG when the patient has his mouth closed.

❖   Explain to the patient that: (1) He must brush the ONG to keep it clean; it can gather tartar just like natural teeth. (2) When he is not using it, leave it in a container filled with water, otherwise it may shrink slightly and not fit well. (3) If he leaves it out of the water and it shrinks slightly, put it in water for a while and it should expand and fit again.

Chapter 14

TREATMENT DENTURE (FLIPPER)

❖ Just as in all other prosthetic treatment, use a quality dental laboratory. The flipper will be aesthetic and require less adjustment.

❖ Explain to the patient that a flipper is a temporary treatment and is done for aesthetic purposes only. Tell him he should remove it to eat and that he will have to get adjusted to speaking with it. Warn the patient that the flipper may last up to 6 months but may break before if he is not careful in its use.

❖ Warn the patient that a flipper in the lower arch can be difficult to use. It can be uncomfortable and does not function well for eating.

❖ A flipper replacing one or more maxillary teeth can be U shaped in order not to interfere excessively with tongue movement. If the tooth is an incisor, often a small U-shaped denture base going from premolar to premolar is enough to provide support and stability. If the base is relined with Coe-Soft (GC Corporation, Tokyo, Japan) upon delivery, there can be enough retention to the point where no clasps are needed.

Chapter 15

COMPLETE DENTURE

Replacing a Complete Denture – Prior to Starting Treatment

❖ Determine whether the patient really needs a new complete denture (CD). Sometimes, when the denture is only two or three years old, a reline will suffice. Check the condition of the teeth and of the denture base. Check retention (good retention—does not come out easily), stability (good stability—there is only slight lateral movement), and support (good support—only slight movement when gently pushed against the alveolar ridge).

❖ Evaluate the health of the denture bearing area. When the denture bearing area is inflamed, often it is due to a fungal infection caused by the patient not cleaning his dentures properly and/or sleeping with them on. Teach him how to clean his denture—brush the denture with non-abrasive soap and a soft brush, immerse it in 0.5 % NaOCl solution for no more than 10 minutes a day until the inflammation resolves— and teach him to always sleep without the dentures.[1] Usually this treatment will suffice for the inflammation to resolve. If the inflammation persists after the patient is given these instructions, prescribe him an antifungal agent.[2]

Note: The reason not to immerse the CD in a stronger concentration of NaOCl, and for longer periods of time, is because it may eventually cause discoloration of the prosthesis.

❖ Determine whether the alveolar ridge has adequate height and width to provide retention. When examining the patient, feel the alveolar ridge with your fingers. Occasionally, especially on the

---

1 Porta S, Lucena-Ferreira S, Silva W, Cury A. Evaluation of sodium hypochlorite as a denture cleanser: a clinical study. *Gerodontology* Volume 32, Issue 4, pages 260–266, December 2015.
2 Allen P, McCarthy S. *Complete Dentures: From Planning to Problem Solving.* 2nd Edition, 2012, pages 27 – 30. Quintessence Publishing Co. Ltd.

maxillary anterior area, visually the alveolar ridge may appear to be adequate, but tactile examination will reveal it to be soft and compressible. The underlying bone having been resorbed and the ridge consisting mainly of soft tissue. When this is the case, this portion of the ridge will not provide retention, stability, or support to the denture.

❖   Ask the patient if he has had many dentures and for how long he has had his present denture. If the patient has not had many dentures, or if he has had the present one for many years, there is a good chance he will be satisfied with the treatment you render. If the patient comes with a little bag full of dentures (all the dentures that were made for him and that don't fit) and starts complaining about his previous dentist, beware! You may be better off referring him to a prosthodontist. The prosthodontist will be better prepared to treat this case.

❖   If the patient has had the same CD for many years and is pleased with the shape and arrangement of its teeth, ask him if he would like the teeth in the new denture to look similar to his present one. If so, make an impression of the CD and have the lab make the tooth set-up as similar as possible to the model of the present CD. This will greatly increase the probability of the patient being pleased with his new prosthesis.

Reasons for Referring to a Prosthodontist

Choose the case carefully. If you see that there is a possibility that the patient may not be satisfied with the treatment, refer him to a prosthodontist. The following are my reasons for referring. Perhaps the reader will feel comfortable and be successful treating some of the cases I would have referred.

❖   Reasons for referring a CUD: (1) palatine torus; (2) overly demanding patient; (3) inadequate alveolar ridge (very resorbed or with severe undercuts).

❖   Reasons for referring for a CLD: (1) overly demanding patient; (2) anything less than an ideal alveolar ridge.

Complete Upper Denture – Prior to Starting

❖   If the patient presents for extraction of all the remaining maxillary teeth and fabrication of a CUD, consider as the treatment of choice an immediate <u>temporary</u> denture instead of an immediate <u>definitive</u> denture. Fabricate a definitive CUD 4 to 6 months after the extractions, when the soft and hard tissues have stabilized. A CUD, fabricated 4 to 6 months after extractions, will usually be better fitting, more aesthetic and more comfortable than an immediate definitive denture delivered at the day of extractions, with a hard reline done 4 to 6 months later. At the day of the extractions, reline the temporary denture with Coe-soft (GC Corporation, Tokyo, Japan) and deliver it after adjusting the occlusion. Replace the reline two to four times as necessary during the four- to six-month period, as the soft and hard tissues heal and change shape. Explain to the patient that the denture bearing area will shrink as the tissues heal and, as a result, the prosthesis will become loose. When this occurs, he must come in for a new reline to improve denture retention. Consider not charging for the soft relines as this is part of the overall treatment.

❖   Occasionally, an older patient will present with a full-arch FPD which is loose due to carious, non-restorable abutments, and which must be replaced by a CD or an implant supported prosthesis. Prior to starting, ask the patient if he would like the teeth of the new prosthesis to look similar to his FPD. If so, send a model of the FPD to the lab and keep another copy. Have the lab make the immediate temporary denture tooth set up as similar to patient's FPD as possible. Send the model of the FPD to the lab again, together with the jaw relation registration, when it is time to do the tooth wax up of the definitive CUD.

CUD - Tips for Taking the Impression

❖   Take a good study model impression. Do it yourself, instead of having the assistant do it. Perform border mold movements as you take the alginate impression.

❖   When preparing the model for fabrication of the custom tray, relieve with wax only the undercuts. The closer the tray fits to the tissues, the better. Light Cured Triad (Dentsply, York, PA) is a quick and easy to use material, good for making custom trays.

❖   When trying in the custom tray for a CUD impression, place your finger at the center of the tray (middle of the palate) and do border mold movements, that is, with your free hand pull the lip and cheeks down, towards the tray. If the tray moves down when you pull on the soft tissues, it means the border in that section of the tray is overextended. You must then reduce that section of the tray by grinding. Repeat this process until there is no more downward movement of the tray when border mold movements are done.

❖   Border mold with compound in 4 sections: anterior, lateral borders one at a time, and posterior. Use green compound. If you wet your glove in the hot water you are using for the border mold procedure, you can touch the softened compound to shape it in the way you want, without it sticking to your gloved fingers. Pull the soft tissue down for each section done. Tell the patient to relax his lips and to open his mouth just enough to allow you room to work. Have the patient move his mandible laterally, to the right and left sides, when border molding the maxillary tuberosity areas. When border molding the posterior area, close the patient's nostrils with your fingers and have him attempt to blow air through his nose.

❖   After border molding: (1) The tray must have retention. If it does not, this lack of retention may be transferred to the CUD. Redo the border molding until it has some retention, that is, until the tray offers some resistance when you pull it down. (2) The tray must not become loose when you pull on the soft tissues. If it becomes loose when you pull on the soft tissues, this means that the compound is overextended. This overextension will likely be transferred to the CUD. Soften the compound in the area corresponding to where it became loose when you pulled and redo the border molding movements.

❖   Consider using a polysulfide impression material for the final impression. This material has a long setting time which allows you to capture the soft tissue positions when you do the border molding movements. On the downside, it has an unpleasant smell, and it distorts quickly after it has set. Before taking the impression, warn the patient that the material you are using does not have the most pleasant of odors. Let him smell it before you put it in his mouth. This way, he will be prepared and will not be negatively surprised. Within ½ an hour of taking the impression, pour it in stone, in other words, make the mastercast. Within this time frame, distortion will not yet have affected your impression. Keep in mind that the mastercast is not done by simply pouring the impression. Prior to pouring, the impression must be prepared with wax so that the mucobuccal folds will be reproduced in stone.

❖   When taking the final impression, spread the material to an even thickness over the entire impression surface of the tray and over the compound at its borders. Place it in the mouth and apply moderate force at the center of the tray with your index finger while doing border mold movements with the other hand. Every minute or so, for the first four minutes, clamp the patient's nostrils shut and have the patient attempt to blow air through his nose. This will improve the seal on the posterior border of the impression. Perform the border mold movements, while applying steady finger pressure to the center of the impression tray with the other hand, for the duration of the seven minutes it takes for the material to set completely.

❖   Upon removal of the tray, inspect the impression carefully. The impression material must evenly cover the tray and the compound at its borders. If the impression material does not cover the denture bearing area completely, or if there are bubbles, the impression should be repeated.

CUD - Tips for Jaw Relations Registration

❖ First, adjust the lip support surface of the wax rim. Remove wax (or add if necessary) so that the lip is resting in a normal, comfortable, and aesthetic position (neither too far forward, nor too far back).

❖ Adjusting the vertical height of the anterior portion of the maxillary wax rim: In most patients, especially if it is an older person, it looks more natural if the upper lip covers the incisal edges when the patient is at rest with the mouth slightly open than if tooth structure shows at this same position. The anterior portion of the maxillary wax rim should be adjusted so that it is hidden by a relaxed upper lip. When the wax rim is placed at this height, it is very likely that there will be adequate freeway space.

❖ When you are finished adjusting the maxillary wax rim check phonetics: (1) Check the S sounds. Have the patient count from 60 to 65 and say Mississippi a couple of times. The lower teeth should not touch the upper wax rim. There should be 1 to 2 mm space between them when the S sound is produced. If the lower teeth touch the upper wax rim, the wax should be reduced in height. (2) Check the V sounds. The "incisal edge" of the maxillary wax rim should touch the wet line of the lower lip.

❖ A way to mark the midline on the wax rim: Have the patient hold a dental floss at the center of his forehead (place the floss there and help the patient place his finger over it). With one hand hold the floss down the middle of his face (which does not always coincide with the middle of the nose) and with the other hand, using a sharp-edged instrument, mark the wax rim where the floss is.

❖ A way to register the bite: Carve non-parallel V-shaped 2 mm to 3 mm deep grooves on the posterior occlusal surface of the wax rim(s) and have the patient bite down on the bite registration material that you use for crown and bridge.

CUD - Tips for Tooth Wax-up Try In

❖   Place denture adhesive on the denture base before inserting it in the patient's mouth to obtain retention so that you can better check phonetics.

❖   Let the patient know that the only thing that will remain the same are the teeth and the way they are set up. Sometimes, at the tooth wax up try-in, a patient will get anxious, say that the denture is uncomfortable or a little loose, because he believes that the acrylic base where the teeth are set is the definitive treatment. By explaining the above to the patient before inserting the tooth wax up in the patient's mouth, you will reduce his level of anxiety.

❖   When checking aesthetics, give a mirror to the patient and let him decide for himself whether he likes the tooth set up. It is better not to say it looks good before he has his say. Remain quiet and let him make up his mind on his own. If the patient states halfheartedly that he likes it, try to find out what is displeasing to him. If the patient is satisfied but you see there is something that can clearly be improved, such as too much tooth structure showing when he smiles, or the denture midline not coinciding with the patient's midline, explain your opinion to the patient and send the case back to the lab for adjustment. It is important to keep in mind that the additional time you and the patient will spend in this case is nothing compared to the years of more aesthetic service he will get from the corrected tooth set up. If the patient asks your opinion and you think it looks good, tell him so.

❖   Have the patient count from 60 to 65 and say Mississippi twice. During the S sounds ask the patient if he feels the teeth touch. Look to see if they touch. If they do, send the case back to the lab to close the bite. You can write in the instruction something like: "Please close the bite 2 mm at central incisors."

❖   Check V and F sounds. If the F sounds like V, anterior maxillary teeth may be too long. If the V sounds like F, the teeth may be too short.

❖   Use excellent quality acrylic teeth. They are more expensive but also more aesthetic and more resistant to wear and discoloration than cheaper teeth. The goal is for the patient to have this denture for many years and the teeth to remain aesthetic for this length of time.

CUD - Tips for the Delivery Appointment:

❖ Let the patient decide for himself whether he likes the denture. Just as in the tooth wax up try-in, it is better not to say, "The denture looks great," before the patient has his say. Instead, you can give him a mirror and say, "Take a look please and see how you like it." If he asks your opinion, tell him what you think.

❖ Check retention, stability, and support.

❖ Take your time adjusting the occlusion. A proper occlusion increases patient comfort and improves retention.

❖ Explain to the patient about denture care. Remind the patient that he must take the denture off to sleep. Explain why (he may develop a fungal infection on the denture bearing area if he sleeps with it).

❖ Advise the patient that sore spots will likely develop and that he must come in for denture adjustment. Explain that if he does not come in, the sore spots may become ulcerations.

❖ Schedule a follow-up visit for the following day after delivery to check for sore spots. Have the patient wear the denture constantly during the first 24 hours (not remove them to sleep) so that you may clearly see any sore spots which may have developed.

❖ If you see that, for whatever reason, the CUD you fabricated is not adequate, fabricate a new one at no charge to the patient.

❖ When there is no retention, a reline may give it retention. One can try a soft reline at first to see if there is improvement. If there is, the dental laboratory can convert the soft reline into a permanent reline.

Complete Lower Denture

❖ For a CLD consider warning the patient that it may be difficult to function with it. It will likely take longer for him to adapt to it than to a

CUD. If you see that the alveolar ridge is less than ideal, consider referring the patient to a prosthodontist.

❖ Occasionally a patient presents with extensive caries and/or advanced periodontal disease in the lower arch. Often, in these cases, the canines, sometimes along with one or two premolars, are the only teeth with adequate bone support or that are restorable. When faced with this situation, consider leaving the canines (and premolars) in order to provide retention and stability to the lower prosthesis until these teeth are lost or until the patient is ready for an implant treatment. One can fabricate the prosthesis taking the same steps as if it were a CLD. The main difference is that the custom tray must be fabricated with compartments for the remaining teeth. When making the final impression, light-bodied Permalastic (Kerr, Orange, CA) is placed in the "canine compartments," and regular Permalastic (Kerr, Orange, CA) is placed on the denture bearing area. The finished case may have wrought wire clasps around the canines. Later, when the patient loses the remaining teeth (which may take months or years to happen), the missing teeth can be easily added to the prosthesis by the dental laboratory, converting it into a CLD. The disadvantage of this treatment is the expense and additional visits required for eventually adding the teeth to the denture.

As in all other prosthodontic treatments, it is important to explain to the patient the advantages and disadvantages of this alternative treatment. Part of the explanation can be: "If we can keep the canines, they will provide some retention to the lower denture and make it easier for you to eat and speak than if the denture is only supported by your gums. Later, when you lose these teeth, we can add them to the prosthesis."

When the patient is ready, the same prosthesis can be converted into an implant retained overdenture.

❖ A very good option for restoring an edentulous mandible seems to be the All-on-4 treatment. A 10 year follow up study published in 2011 showed it has more than 90% success rate for the implants individually, and 99% success rate for the prosthesis.[3] The treatment consists in four implants placed in the mandible and immediately restored with an implant supported prosthesis. The distal implants are placed anterior to the mental foramen, but in a distally inclined position, to reduce the cantilever arm of the prosthesis.

3 Malo P, et al. A longitudinal study of the survival of All-on-4 implants in the mandible with up to 10 years of follow-up. *J Am Dent Assoc.* 2011 Mar;142(3):310-20

Chapter 16

REMOVABLE PARTIAL DENTURE

Selecting the Case

❖   If the patient already has an RPD, ask him for how long he has had it and determine if it needs to be replaced. If it is just a tooth that fractured off and the remaining structure fits well and is in good shape, instead of making a new RPD it is better to repair the present RPD.

❖   In my experience, RPDs with tooth anchored precision attachments do not work very well. It is common to have some form of failure happen not too long after placement. In most cases where tooth replacement is needed, the best treatment option is an implant supported restoration. If the patient is concerned enough about aesthetics to pay the extra cost and undergo the additional treatment required for an RPD with tooth anchored precision attachments, then, clearly, implants are a much more appropriate treatment. Explain this to your patient. Consider referring him to a prosthodontist if he insists on having tooth anchored precision attachments.

Prior to Starting the Treatment

❖   Warn the patient that: (1) there will be metal clasps, and these often can be seen when the patients speaks or smiles; (2) the RPD will have to be removed at night before going to sleep.

❖   While discussing the treatment with the patient, if you are unsure whether a clasp will be visible when he smiles, it is better to tell him that it will likely show when he smiles. This way he will not be disappointed if it does and will be pleased if it doesn't.

❖   In order to better illustrate to the patient what the clasp will look like, place an instrument of similar shape and dimension, such as a spoon excavator, at the same position on the tooth as the clasp will be.

Have the patient look in the mirror as he does a forced smile so that he can see the instrument on his tooth.

❖   Prior to starting the RPD treatment, make sure there is no remaining caries, active periodontal disease or necrotic pulps. If you detect any of these once you have already started, the initial treatment plan will be affected. Also, it will increase the cost of the treatment. It is always a negative surprise to the patient when he finds out he will have to pay more than he was originally told.

❖   At the initial visit, take alginate impressions for the fabrication of study models. Survey the model of the arch that will be treated with an RPD and draw on it a detailed design of the RPD. At the next visit, show the study model with the design to the patient. Remind him that you will have to grind his teeth a little in preparation for the RPD. Show him where the rests will be. If a cingulum rest is planned, warn him that he may feel the groove with his tongue when he is not using the RPD but that normally one gets used to it. What can also be done, to better illustrate your explanation, is to prepare the occlusal and cingulum rests on the study model with the bur while the patient watches. This will make it easier for the patient to understand what you are talking about. The more he knows what to expect, the more at peace he will be with the treatment.

❖   If there is a choice between an I-bar clasp assembly and a circumferential clasp assembly, the I-bar seems to be the better option. It is less visible, and on distal extension RPDs, it transmits less torqueing forces to the supporting tooth.

❖   On a distal extension RPD, if the abutment is a crowned premolar, it may be better not to place a clasp assembly on it. A clasp assembly in this case (where there is movement of the prosthesis when the patient eats) may gradually loosen the crown and pull it out, sometimes along with the post if there is one. Therefore, on a distal extension RPD, if possible, it may be better to skip the crowned tooth and place the clasp assembly on the next tooth.

❖   Draw the design you choose not only on the surveyed study model but also on the laboratory prescription. Besides drawing the RPD, give clear written instructions of how you want it made. Include the surveyed study model in the package to the laboratory.

❖   A great book to help in the design of RPDs is *Atlas of Removable Partial Denture Design* by Dr. Russell J. Straton and Dr. Frank J. Wiebelt, Quintessence Books.

Fabricating the RPD

❖   Use high quality acrylic teeth and do a wax up try-in, even if you are only replacing a couple of posterior teeth on a tooth supported RPD. If, for some reason, there was a mistake along the way and the teeth are out of occlusion, it is easier to adjust while the teeth are set on wax then after the case is finished. The wax try-in also makes it simpler to make changes if the patient is not satisfied with the aesthetics of the tooth set up.

RPD Delivery

❖   When delivering the RPD, give the instructions on RPD care yourself, instead of having the assistant do it. Remind the patient again that he must remove it to sleep. Tell him that if sore spots develop, he must come in immediately for adjustment of the RPD. Schedule a follow-up appointment for the next day before dismissing the patient.

Chapter 17

OFFICE MANAGEMENT

General Tips

❖ Consider using always quality materials and a quality dental laboratory. This seems to go against the "watch the overhead" maxim but, in the long run, it is really an investment which will likely increase your income and bring about the personal fulfillment of doing one's best for the patient. The better the materials and dental laboratory, the better the quality of the treatment one provides and the longer it will last. As a consequence of providing a lasting, aesthetic treatment, you will have a satisfied patient who will return to your office and who will, for years to come, refer other patients. The increase in cost resultant from using quality materials and dental laboratory will be offset by a consistently full schedule.

❖ If your office is not paperless, have a good, simple filing system, with all the charts in one place, well filed and easily accessible. If filing is done carelessly, your staff can spend precious time looking for a misfiled chart.

❖ The more organized the office is, each item in its proper place, from burs to front desk supplies, the more smoothly the day will go, the more quickly things will get done.

❖ Consider using digital radiography in your practice. It is not a basic need (such as is a dental management software) because film radiography works very well and produces excellent images. However, digital radiography has some advantages over film radiography which make it worth the investment. Digital radiography produces images immediately as opposed to taking several minutes to be developed, and with a much lower dose of radiation to the patient than film radiography. In addition, the software allows the image to be enhanced, such as altering brightness and contrast in order to improve visibility of an anatomical feature or lesion, and measured, such as when doing a root canal.

❖ Advertise at first. Once the schedule is full and there is a steady flow of new patients referred by other patients, consider stopping advertising. If the schedule is full, there is no need for the marketing expense.

❖ Consider making it a part of your daily routine to arrive at the dental office at least a half hour before the first appointment so that you have time to: (1) Make sure everything is in order in the office. (2) Review your last entry in the chart of each of the patients of record (i.e., those who are not first-time patients) that will be seen that day and go over their medical histories. This will refresh your memory as to the details of the last treatment rendered, as to the patient's general oral health, and will remind you of any red flags regarding a medical condition. By reviewing the charts, when you walk into the operatory with the awaiting patient, you will walk into a familiar and comfortable situation.

Office Layout

❖ Consider not having a TV in the waiting room. Not everyone wants to watch the same program and some people do not want to watch TV at all. Some interesting, illustrated books and magazines are all that is needed to keep the patient entertained during his time there, if he does not feel like using his mobile device.

❖ In the operatory, have the patient chair facing a window or a glass wall, if possible, with a garden on the other side. This will create a much more pleasant atmosphere for the patient than if the operatory is a windowless room with no view of the outside.

❖ Set up the operatories in a way that the cabinets are within easy reach of the assistant while leaving her plenty of room to move around. This will make it quick and easy for her to get what is needed during treatment. On your side of the chair, make sure there is also plenty of room for you to move. Neither you nor the assistant should be in a cramped, uncomfortable space. You will spend a good part of your day there and you should be comfortable.

❖   If you are a Christian, consider placing a small picture of the Holy Family, or a small Crucifix or Cross, in the operatory, at a location where your eyes will most easily rest when you are sitting in your stool, ready to begin work. This is an unobtrusive reminder to you that, God is above all; that He is watching you and your patient with loving eyes and that He wants you to do your best for him.

Fee Management

❖   Charge a fair price. Not too high, not too low. If the fee is too high, the patient may feel cheated when he finds out other dentist's fees. If it is too low, it may be difficult for you to meet the office overhead. In the later instance, to compensate for the lower income, you may have to lower your expenses by hiring employees at lesser wages, using lower quality materials, and performing treatment in less time. As a result, the quality of care will likely decrease, and with it, patient satisfaction.

❖   Charge everyone the same. Patients talk to each other, and it will be an unpleasant surprise for one if he finds out he has paid more than his friend for the same treatment.

❖   Generally, consider not giving discounts. Instead, depending on the case, one can offer a free cleaning, or not charge for an exam or X-ray. If you give a patient a discount, his friends may hear about it and ask for a fee reduction, and then will feel cheated if you don't give it. This is a guideline that provides for a more peaceful running of your practice.

❖   For root canal therapy (RCT), charge by type of tooth and not by number of canals, that is, charge for anterior, premolar and molar. This way, the cost of treatment will not change if you find an additional canal, or if there is one canal less than expected. You and your patient have already agreed on a fee before you start the procedure, it makes life simpler to stick to this fee.

❖ Have one single fee for crowns, independent of which material you use and of what the lab fees are. Charge the same fee whether it is an all-porcelain crown, porcelain fused to metal (PFM) or gold. This will encourage the patient to choose the crown that is best for his case. Price will not be a factor in his choice.

❖ Treatment plan well and make as accurate an estimate of the cost as possible. This will reduce the number of occasions, once the treatment has already started, in which the patient will have to be told that the cost will be higher than expected. It can be disappointing for the patient to find out he will have to pay more than what he was first told.

❖ The patient must know what he will be expected to pay at the day of the appointment before any treatment is performed. As in the point above, no one likes to be surprised by an unexpected fee.

❖ Teach the front desk person and assistants that before passing a patient into the operatory for an emergency, they must inform him that there will be a fee for the exam and X-rays even if no treatment is rendered. It is your time, materials used in making a diagnosis, and hard-earned knowledge, and you deserve to be paid for it. If you spend only a few minutes with the patient, you have the option of, after seeing him, charging only for the X-ray.

❖ One of the ways in which a practice can lose income is when treatments rendered go unpaid. To prevent this, when it is a cash patient, have the front desk person advise him that the treatment must be paid in full on the day it is done. If it is a procedure that takes more than one visit to finish, such as a prosthesis or some root canal therapies, the payments can be divided by the number of visits required to complete it. If it takes two visits, the patient makes two equal payments, one at each visit. Three visits, three payments.

Billing the Insurance

❖ In order to avoid exceeding the insurance companies' frequency clause (the insurance covers a procedure only if a certain amount of time has passed since it was last performed) both you and the front desk person should be on the lookout for possible traps. The two most common infringements of this clause that occur in the day to day of a dental office are a prophylaxis done before 6 months have passed since the last one and a prosthesis, including crowns, being replaced before the stipulated number of years have passed since the prior placement.

To avoid performing a prophylaxis before it will be covered by the insurance, when scheduling an appointment for this procedure the staff must check the patient's records to make sure that six months have passed since his last cleaning.

To avoid an insurance denial for a prosthetic replacement, have the front desk person send a pretreatment authorization form to the insurance company. Start the treatment only after you have received a response, and the patient has been informed of how much he will have to pay. This can range from the full amount, if the insurance states treatment is not covered, to no payment on the part of the patient, if the insurance covers the whole fee.

❖   Some indemnity insurance plans are very reliable in their coverage of the initial placement of a prosthesis. Others not so much. In the latter case, one may send a claim for a crown or a removable partial denture (RPD) and get a denial of payment in return or be paid a small percentage of the amount billed. Therefore, it may be prudent to send a pretreatment estimate for every prosthetic case until one learns which insurance companies are reliable and which are not.

❖   When sending a pretreatment estimate to an insurance company, consider always including a copy of the X-rays of the area being treated (for an RPD, a copy of the panoramic X-ray). In the long run, this saves time. If X-rays are not sent, often the insurance company will request them to determine if the treatment is covered. This exchange can add at least a couple of weeks for an answer to be given.

Hygiene Management

❖   Consider allowing one hour for cleaning appointments, instead of 45 minutes, and one hour and thirty minutes for scaling and root planning (SC and RP) two quadrants. This will give the hygienist more time to provide an unhurried, thorough, quality prophylaxis to the patient, and to keep his/her operatory clean and tidy.

❖   Once the hygienist is finished with the prophylaxis on a new patient, he can be passed to another operatory and one of the assistants can take the FMX. This frees the hygiene chair for another cleaning.

❖   The hygiene recall card! This is a valuable tool that assists in keeping the hygiene schedule full. Before dismissing his/her patient, the hygienist gives a recall card for him to fill out. The patient simply enters his name and address, and he/she then files it with all the other cards filled out during that month. Five months later, he/she will mail the group of cards filled out that month. The card is a reminder to the patient that it is time to schedule an appointment for a cleaning. It can say something like this: "A friendly reminder from your hygienist that it is time to schedule your appointment." There are several different recall cards available through dental supply outlets. Some with jokes, some with a beautiful scene of nature, etc. Have a few different types at hand and let the patient choose the one he likes.

Provide the hygienist with a filing box. Within it should be 12 folders, one for each month. The cards are filed in the folder for the 5th month after the day of the cleaning. For example: if the cleaning was in January, the card must be filed in the folder for June. When June arrives, already in the first week he/she mails the cards that are stored in the June folder. The patients that call in response to schedule are then given appointments for the month of July, six months after their cleaning in January.

Chapter 18

INTERACTION WITH PATIENTS

❖ Educate your patient. Explain to him the condition that he has and its probable causes, be it caries, a non-restorable tooth, periodontal disease, non-carious cervical lesions, etc. Teach how to prevent this condition from occurring again. Explain all the treatment options, their risks and benefits. An educated patient will better understand the condition he has and will be more motivated to take the necessary steps to prevent it from happening again. He will probably take better care of his teeth, in which case your treatment will last much longer.

❖ Be always kind and understanding with your patients. Try to look at the situation from their point of view.

❖ Generally, if a patient wants to sell you goods or a service, do not buy it or accept it. If you do, it may interfere with your relationship with him as a patient. Sometimes the service or good is inadequate, or you decide you don't want it anymore. This may cause some tension between you and the patient.

❖ If the patient has poor oral hygiene (OH), do not be overbearing when you tell him about it. One way to tell the patient he has poor OH without hurting his feelings is, "You have very good teeth, but your oral hygiene can improve a little." Give the patient a handheld mirror and ask him to look while you show him the plaque on his teeth. You can scrape it off with the explorer and say something like, "See, you have a little plaque here. This can cause gingivitis and cavities."

❖ When discussing prosthodontic treatments with the patient, show him models with the different cases you are talking about. Have a clear (transparent) model with implants so that he can visualize what you are explaining to him. Have RPDs, complete dentures, the different types of crowns, fixed partial dentures (FPDs) and treatment dentures (flippers) available to show to the patient. It is much easier for him to understand the treatment if he can see what you are talking about.

❖   When you notice that the patient is a demanding person, with high expectations, it is prudent to realistically lower his expectations before he invests time, money, and effort into a treatment. In this way, if he opts to have the treatment done, it is less likely that he will be disappointed with the outcome.

❖   Do not worry if a patient decides not to do a treatment because you presented a realistic, though unpromising, picture to him. He is entitled to make an informed decision. St Augustine wrote: "The truth is like a lion, just let it out and it will take care of itself." It is better to perform no treatment than to paint a rosy, unrealistic picture to a patient to "sell a case." When this happens, the lion of truth will come back to bite the dentist in the form of a disappointed, frustrated patient when the treatment fails to meet his expectations.

❖   At each visit, the patient should be clearly informed of the procedure being done that day. Always, before starting a treatment, before even administering the anesthesia, give a hand mirror to the patient and show him which tooth you are going to treat on that visit. (Teach the assistant to keep this mirror clean. The patient can get a bad impression if he can't see his reflection clearly because of a dirty mirror.)

❖   Do not contradict the patient outright. No one likes to be contradicted. Let the patient have his say and then explain to him the facts. Do so humbly, without an attitude of superiority. Saint Augustine wrote, "There is something in humility which strangely exalts the heart." Hopefully, your humble attitude will exalt your patient's heart and he will be at peace with your treatment recommendation. If the patient insists in his point of view and he is wrong but this does not affect the treatment, go on with the procedure. If, however, it does affect the treatment, refer the patient to a specialist and let the specialist know the reason for the referral.

❖   Before you perform a treatment, if you tell the patient the possible negative outcomes, such as, "The tooth may become sensitive and end up needing root canal therapy," or, "The acrylic tooth on this treatment denture may fracture off," the patient will see it as a warning. From the patient's point of view, you will not be held accountable if the warning comes true (remember to always make a notation in the chart of what you tell the patient). If, on the other hand, you wait until the negative outcome occurs to explain why it happened, the patient may see it as an excuse, even though it is not your fault. He may not voice his displeasure, but in his mind, he may blame you for the adverse outcome.

❖   Avoid using the word "permanent" when referring to dental treatment, such as, permanent crown, or permanent cement. No restoration or prosthesis can be thought of as permanent. They may last a very long time, some may last the patient's lifetime, but most eventually will need to be replaced. Therefore, use instead the word "definitive," such as, definitive crown, definitive cement. By using the word definitive instead of permanent, you keep the patient from the false notion that his treatment will never need to be replaced.

❖   Try as much as possible not to keep patients waiting—either on the chair or in the waiting room. There may be someone in this world who likes to wait but I still haven't met him or her. If you notice you will run late, have the assistant call the next patient and the one after him, if necessary, to let him (them) know you are running late. Tell him (them) to come a ½ hour later than his (their) scheduled time. Work through lunch if necessary to make up the time, but avoid as much as you can, running behind schedule. The patient's time is as valuable as your own and he may view the entire treatment in a negative light after having had to wait for an hour to be seen.

If you are running late and the patient is already in the waiting room, ask the front desk person to let him know the amount of time you will be late so that he may use it to go out to stretch his legs or to have a cup of coffee.

❖   It is better not to tell the patient, after you have administered anesthesia, that he will only feel pressure. This is incorrect. He may very well feel pain, not pressure, if the anesthesia does not completely anesthetize the tooth. Pain and pressure are two very different things. Pain, depending on its intensity, can be very distressing. Pressure is at the most a nuisance. Therefore, instead of telling the patient he will only feel pressure, it is better to ask him to let you know if he feels any pain while you work.

Imagine a patient clearly wincing in pain in the chair during treatment, and, instead of stopping, the dentist just keeps on drilling while the assistant yells over the drill noise, "Don't worry, you are just feeling pressure." If the poor patient has the option of going to another dentist, chances are that he will do so.

❖   Write a thorough chart. Make note of what you said to the patient and what he said to you. The chart is a legal document which can protect you in case of litigation. In fact, a detailed entry in the chart can prevent litigation by clearing up any misunderstanding with the patient when a negative situation first occurs. For example, a patient may present with a non-restorable fracture on a maxillary premolar after RCT was performed by you on the tooth. He will be understandably upset to lose the tooth but, in addition, he may blame you for the loss. By reminding him that, before doing the RCT, you explained the necessity of restoring the tooth with a crown soon after RCT was performed, in order to avoid risking the loss of the tooth due to a fracture, and showing him the detailed entry in his records to prove it (something like, "Prior to starting RCT, pt was advised tooth needs to be restored with a crown, or it may fracture within days. Pt advised to eat soft foods until crown is placed."), there is a good chance he will remember your warning and stop blaming you for the adverse situation.

Note: In digital charts, the software allows one to customize entries such as the one above, where a simple click of the mouse will place it on the patient's records. With handwritten charts one can use abbreviations such as pt, instead of patient, and Cr instead of crown, to speed up the entry.

❖   Do not impose any treatment on your patient. Let him decide if he wants it done. If the patient does not want a treatment, do not insist. If the patient has an antagonistic attitude which does not change after you discuss the matter with him, consider referring him to someone else. Always make notations in the chart when a patient declines a treatment and let the dentist, to whom you referred the patient, know the reason for the referral.

❖   When interacting with the patient, just be natural and treat him with kindness and respect coming from the heart. There is no need to be artificially pleasant in an attempt to have the person like you. The quality of your work, the low amount of discomfort the patient feels when being treated by you, the efficient, kind and respectful staff, are what will win you his confidence.

Chapter 19

EMPLOYEE MANAGEMENT

❖ Before hiring someone, do a "working interview." Let them work with you one or two days on a trial basis. This is important because it will give you some idea whether you will get along working together. If this person works well, hire them temporarily, that is, without benefits for one or two months. If, after this period, you have no doubt the person is a good worker, hire the person definitively and with benefits. Count the vacation time from the very first day he/she worked. That is, the first day of the working interview.

❖ Make the responsibilities of the employees clear to them when you first hire them. Their duties may be given to them in writing. Let them know, in detail, all that they will be required to do. For example, when explaining his/her duties as a dental assistant: "You will have to clean the office in the morning, on the days when the cleaning person does not come in. You have to clean the sink, the toilet, mop the floor, dust the cabinets, clean the sinks in the operatories, vacuum the floor," etc.

❖ If you have a busy office with a full schedule, have 2 assistants and one front desk person. While one assistant helps you with the treatment you are performing, the other assistant can: (1) Work on another patient, such as: make a temporary crown, take alginate impressions, take X-rays on an emergency patient, etc. (2) Answer phone calls. (3) Call patients to confirm the following day's appointments or to fill the schedule in case there is a cancellation. (4) Call insurance companies to verify patient benefits. (5) Order supplies.

❖ Teach the assistants how to work the front desk. If the front desk person takes a vacation or is ill and cannot come to work, one of the assistants can temporarily take up her duties as a backup.

❖ Ideally, the front desk person should have experience as a dental assistant. In this way if one of the assistants does not come in for work, or is busy with another project, the front desk person can help you with the treatment being done.

❖ Check the payments every day, no matter how honest your employees may be. Let your employees see you doing it. This is a theft deterrent because it greatly reduces the temptation to steal.

❖ Treat your employees the way you would want to be treated. Be kind and respectful. Pay competitive wages and give good benefits: paid lunch time, medical insurance, retirement fund, paid holidays, paid sick days, increase the vacation time in proportion to the number of years the employee has worked at your office. After having assured yourself that the employee is a conscientious and hard worker it is fair to reward him/her accordingly. By giving the employees good benefits, they will feel valued and will be more at peace and happy with their jobs. This translates into a pleasant, relaxed environment in your office. A pleasant, relaxed atmosphere, in turn, is attractive to the patients and benefits you also. You will get up in the morning looking forward to getting to work and spending the day there.

❖ Do not waste time with an employee who turns out to be lazy. Let him/her go.

Responsibilities of the Front Desk Person/Office Manager

❖ Be honest, firm, and efficient.

❖ Create dental claims, bill patients and insurance companies.

❖ Verify insurance. Contact the insurance companies of the patients that will be seen the following day and make sure there is enough benefit left to cover the treatments that will be rendered. If a prosthesis is to be started and a pretreatment estimate was sent to the insurance company, make sure the response with the amount the insurance will pay has been received.

Verifying the insurance is an important guideline to be followed. It is not good practice to find out that the insurance does not cover a treatment only after it is already completed. If this happens, you have the option of billing the patient. However, nobody likes receiving an unexpected bill. The patient may feel cheated or feel that your office is disorganized. If you don't bill the patient, you have the loss of overhead cost for that hour of work without an income.

❖   When an active patient schedules for a cleaning and an exam, look at his treatment history to make sure enough time has passed since the last visit for the insurance to cover the treatment.

❖   Create a list of overdue dental claims. Much income can be lost through dental claims that go unpaid. The dental claim that your office creates can get lost in the mail, cyberspace or be the victim of human error somewhere within the insurance company. To prevent this loss, the front desk person should, once a month, create a list of unpaid dental claims that are over two months old. The dental programs available can easily generate this information, that is, create an "aging claims list." The front desk person must then contact the insurance companies and ask why the claims have not been paid. If the reason is that the claim was not received, he/she must send a new claim.

❖   Enter claim denials in patients' ledgers. When insurance companies deny a payment, they will send your office an explanation for the denial. The front desk person must enter this claim denial in the patient's ledger to prevent the claim from appearing in the "aging claims list." You must then decide whether to charge the patient or not. Proper insurance verification prior to starting a treatment will reduce claim denials to a minimum.

❖   Create a thorough "charge sheet" after the schedule for the following day has been confirmed. The "charge sheet" is an important collection tool. It makes it easy for the front desk person to know how much the patient will have to pay. The assistants should also be familiar with it in case they are subbing in for the front desk.

To create a charge sheet:

1) Print a copy of the schedule for the next day, after the appointments have been confirmed.

2) Look at patient's account ledger.

3) Write below his name what his balance is—credit, debit or zero balance

4) If it is a cash patient, write "cash" below or next to the patient's balance.

5) If it is an insurance patient, write "ins" and how much he has left in insurance benefit for that year, such as, "ins - $756.00 left for year". This will allow you to know how much treatment can be done without the patient having to pay out of pocket.

6) If the patient's insurance does not cover the whole cost of the procedure, write what the insurance will pay and how much the patient must pay. The patient must know how much he will have to pay before you begin the treatment.

❖   Know what procedures were performed, and charge accordingly. Occasionally, a different treatment (or an additional treatment) may be performed other than what was originally planned. When this occurs, the front desk person must be aware of the change so that he/she may charge accordingly. To let him/her know of the change, you can do a quick entry in the digital chart with the information and later make a more thorough entry, or you can write it on a sticky note and give it to the assistant to take to the front desk person. Prior to performing a different procedure or an additional one, if the patient has no insurance, it is important that he be told of the cost difference. If he has insurance, you must know whether the benefits he has left for the year are enough to cover the different or additional treatment so that you can inform him of the cost difference.

❖   Print the "daysheet" for the previous day. The "daysheet" is a valuable management tool that shows, among other things, the production, collection, and types of procedures performed the previous day.

❖   Fill any openings in the schedule by calling the patients who need treatment and asking them if they would like to make an appointment.

❖ Make an entry in the patient's chart when he cancels an appointment, fails to come in or is more than 20 minutes late for an appointment.

❖ Charge patients.

❖ Schedule the patient's next appointment before he leaves.

❖ Enter payments in the patient's account ledger.

❖ If one of the assistants is not able to confirm the patients for the next day, confirm the patients himself/herself.

❖ Pull the charts for the next day if the office is not paperless.

❖ Keep front office clean and organized.

❖ Keep an eye on the waiting room. If he/she sees it is messy, organize it. The waiting room is the first impression patients will have when they walk into your office. Hence, it is important that it be neat and pleasant.

❖ Order office supplies.

❖ Keep office machines working such as, replace toner when needed, and add paper to fax and printer.

❖ Wear either scrubs or modest working clothes—no jeans, no short skirts.

❖ Not eat at the front desk. Eating is done in the breakroom. Not chew gum while at the front desk.

❖ Not waste time talking gossip with the patients either on the phone or at the front desk.

❖ If a personal call must be made, not waste time with it.

Responsibilities of the Hygienist:

❖ Be gentle! Have a light hand.

❖ As part of a prophylaxis on an active patient, spot probe mesial and distal of two or three teeth per quadrant; note bleeding upon probing. Write findings in the chart.

❖ When it is an initial exam, do full mouth periodontal probing and note bleeding and mobility. Enter findings in chart. One of the assistants can help with entering the information in the chart.

❖ If a new patient has poor oral hygiene, or a condition that occurs because of poor oral hygiene, such as caries, gingivitis, or periodontal disease, teach the patient how to brush and floss. Have the patient hold a mirror and watch while he/she flosses. Recommend a soft toothbrush and non-abrasive toothpaste to reduce the chances of non-carious cervical lesions forming.

❖ Not be overbearing and negative if the patient has poor oral hygiene. Gently point out that his hygiene can improve. Look for something positive to say along with the fact that hygiene must improve, such as: "You have such nice teeth but there is some plaque, and the gingiva is a little inflamed." Explain consequences of plaque such as gingivitis, caries, and periodontitis. When the hygienist is kind and gentle, it is an added incentive for the patient to follow his/her instructions.

❖ Dab Vaseline on a patient's dry lips prior to starting the prophylaxis. This greatly reduces the patient's discomfort when his lips need to be slightly pulled to have access to posterior teeth.

❖ Take BW X-rays, after scaling and root planning, of the area treated. The hygienist must do this without having to be told. The X-ray is taken to check if interproximal calculus is still present. If the image shows there is interproximal calculus, the hygienist must scale the area again.

❖ Give a recall card to each patient to fill out. File it in the appropriate month folder. The explanation for recall cards can be found on page 149.

❖ Make clear and correct notations in the chart of what he/she is told by you during your examination of his/her patient. That is, make clear notations of your findings and of the treatment needed.

❖ Make clear and correct notations of his/her findings and of the treatment rendered.

❖ Normally the hygienist does not dismiss patients. This is a job for the front desk person and, occasionally, the dental assistant. However, in a busy office, occasionally his/her help may be needed with dismissing his/her patient. If the hygienist dismisses the patient: (1) Ask if he would like to already schedule an appointment for the next cleaning. (2) If there is a dental treatment that needs to be done, schedule an appointment with the dentist. (3) Charge for the treatment rendered if the patient does not have insurance.

❖ If the hygienist has a free hour, such as when a patient cancels an appointment, work on recall. That is, call the patients who are due for a cleaning and ask if they would like to schedule an appointment. Most dental management softwares, if not all, can generate a list of patients who are due for a cleaning in a given month and who are not already scheduled for it.

Responsibilities of the Assistant

Most of the following points can be taught to the assistant after he/she is hired. Ideally, an assistant is hired fresh out of dental assisting school, knowing how to take X-rays and sterilize instruments. In this way, he/she will learn to work in a manner that best fits how you work.

❖ Be kind, gentle and patient.

❖ Clean and sterilize the instruments with care, not in a haphazard manner.

❖ Keep the operatories clean, organized and stocked with supplies. If the assistant sees something on the floor, pick it up. The operatories should be spotless. A dirty, disorganized operatory is unhealthy and gives a bad impression. A spotless operatory assists in creating a pleasant environment for the patient.

❖ Check the patient bathroom a few times a day. Make sure it is clean and stocked. Most patients will be understandably disgusted if they walk into a dirty bathroom at a dental office.

❖ On the days when the cleaning person does not come in: (1) sweep or vacuum all floors; (2) mop operatory and bathroom floors; (3) clean bathroom; (4) organize waiting room.

❖   Know how to: make temporary crowns; place a retraction cord; take good alginate impressions; cement a temporary crown; fabricate bleaching trays, etc. All treatments must be done gently and with concern for the patient's well-being.

❖   Know how to evaluate the quality of an X-ray and have the initiative to retake it if he/she sees that it is inadequate.

❖   While working on the patient, such as placing a retraction cord, ask the patient if he is feeling pain. Call the dentist if the patient is feeling pain.

❖   When alone in the operatory with the patient, if the patient feels like talking, he/she may talk freely and answer any questions he may have. This helps to put the patient at ease. However, when you are in the operatory, you should do the talking and not the assistant. Especially regarding anything treatment related. If you are having a conversation with the patient about the treatment, and the assistant beside you keeps giving his/her input, this may confuse the patient and, also, what you say may carry less weight.

❖   Order dental supplies.

❖   Keep you informed of any necessary equipment repairs or other problem he/she may see.

❖   Know how to work at the front desk, that is: (1) schedule patients; (2) dismiss patients; (3) confirm patients for the following day; (4) charge for treatment performed; (5) verify insurance. With time you can also train the assistant to: (1) enter treatments into dental software and print or email dental claims; (2) prepare day sheet; (3) prepare charge sheet; (4) enter payments in dental software. These last four items normally are responsibilities of the front desk person. However, if this person is absent for any reason, it helps if the assistant knows how to perform them. By training the assistant to do this you are expanding his/her knowledge and preparing him/her to one day become an office manager if he/she so desires.

❖   Confirm the patients for the following day. That is, call them and remind them of their appointment. This should be done in the morning so that, if there are any cancellations, there will be enough time for the front desk person (or the assistant him/herself) to contact other patients and try to fill the schedule.

❖   Answer the phones.

❖   Be punctual.

The Importance of a Quality Staff

It can't be emphasized enough how important it is to have a staff that holds the same work ethic that you do and treats the patients well, for the patients' sake, not because they are supposed to. When the employees enjoy dentistry and are truly concerned for the patient's well-being, their work will be of good quality, and you will have less headaches and less loss in your practice.

❖   Some negative examples of the importance of a quality staff:

-   You prepped a crown and the assistant is now making a temporary. If he/she is rough and heavy handed, it will be unnecessarily uncomfortable to the patient. If the assistant is not careful and fabricates a temporary crown with inadequate margins, open interproximal contacts, poor occlusion, or a rough surface, you or he/she will have to spend valuable time adjusting the temporary crown. It will also be wasted time for the patient.

-   The assistant carelessly fails to see and pick up a bloody gauze sponge that is on the floor, before passing the next patient. When the patient walks into the operatory and sees that gauze on the floor it will give him a negative impression of your office.

-   The assistant fails to order a certain material, such as crown cement, before it runs out. You are ready to cement a crown and there is no permanent cement. You end up having to use a temporary cement instead and having to ask the patient to come back for a second visit to cement the crown with a definitive cement. More wasted time for the patient and for you.

- The assistant fails to follow infection control guidelines and does not wear a mask while taking X-rays or taking an impression. A negative mark, on the patient's mind, regarding your office.

- The hygienist is rough and heavy handed. He/she does not ask if the patient is okay when he/she sees him giving signs of discomfort, and just keeps on working.

- The front desk person inadvertently double books patients.

- The front desk person fails to tell patients the treatment fee before they are passed into the operatory so that they are unpleasantly surprised by an unexpected fee on their way out.

All the examples above are incidents which can happen if the staff is not carefully selected or well trained, and which will drive away patients and their referrals. In addition, such a staff, and the problems that will arise from their work, will create an unpleasant work atmosphere for everyone involved.

On the other hand, when your staff is truly caring and conscientious, when their hearts are into what they are doing, it will create a pleasant environment for the staff themselves, for the patients and for you.

❖   Some positive examples:

- Your assistant, who is polite and has light hands, is making a temporary crown and notices that the patient winces a little bit when he/she places it on the tooth. He/She then immediately stops, asks him if he is okay and lets you know that the patient may be feeling pain.

- Your assistant is making a temporary crown on a maxillary tooth (the tongue is not anesthetized). He/She asks the patient if he feels roughness on the temporary crown with his tongue.

- Every time the patient comes for an appointment, the operatory is clean and neat and the assistant follows infection control procedures to the letter.

- The assistant is gentle when trying on impression trays. If he/she notices signs of discomfort on the patient's face, he/she asks if it is hurting and, if so, tries on another tray.

- The assistant cleans the face of the patient properly after taking an impression with alginate.

- The hygienist is light handed, courteous and truly concerned for the well-being of the patient.

- The front desk person is on top of things. The patients are never surprised by an unexpected bill, are kept well informed about their insurance benefits and there are no scheduling conflicts.

These are very positive ways of the employees conducting themselves which, in addition to your competence, knowledge and skill, will lead to a successful practice.

Chapter 20

A FEW LIFE TIPS

❖ If possible, take a vacation of a couple of weeks once a year. Vacation helps one to recharge the batteries for another year of beautiful dentistry. You can ask a dentist, friend of yours, to take care of the emergency patients for you during this period. When he/she, in turn, goes on vacation, you can return the favor and treat his/her emergency patients.

❖ In the beginning, buy a simple, economic car. Do not pay interest or waste money on a fancy car. This money is better invested in real estate, a retirement fund or in eliminating one's debts. One does not know what the future holds. If, for some reason, something happens and you cannot practice dentistry anymore, being free of debt and perhaps having investments will give you peace of mind.

❖ Do not work too many hours a day. Eight hours a day is plenty. If the office runs well, you can accomplish as much in eight hours as you would in ten hours in a "rocky office." The reason for watching the number of hours you work is because dentistry is a physically demanding profession. If one is not careful, over the years it can take its toll on one's body. You want your back, your eyes, your hearing to be in good shape as you age.

❖ Do not worry about money. It will come if you do good work. Worry instead about providing the best quality treatment that you possibly can to your patient. In this way, your workday will be pleasant and full of accomplishments. A good, quality practice can't help but generate a good income.

❖ This order of priorities leads to a peaceful, happy life: 1st God; 2nd Family; 3rd Work (Dentistry).

Keeping Up to Date

❖   In dentistry new and improved techniques and materials are constantly being developed. Just some years ago, to place a posterior composite restoration was a disservice to the patient due to its poor physical properties. Back then, the material of choice was amalgam. Now, with the improved properties of composites and bonding agents, one can almost say that the opposite is true. Also, not too long ago, if a patient presented with a missing tooth, the best treatment option would have been a fixed partial denture, requiring tooth reduction (often of perfectly healthy teeth) and occasionally requiring RCTs. Now, the treatment of choice is an implant supported restoration which not only leaves adjacent teeth intact, but also possibly helps to preserve the alveolar ridge. Many more examples of recent improvements in all areas of dentistry such as nickel-titanium rotary files, digital radiography, the use of mineral trioxide aggregate in endodontics, can be given. The point here is that one must keep up to date with these new developments to provide the best available treatment to one's patients.

In order to accomplish this, consider creating the habit of studying every day. Peer reviewed dental journals, where the authors have no commercial interest in the materials studied, are good sources of information, as are recently published textbooks. One can have a daily routine of a set hour (early in the morning is great) to study. Belonging to a study group and attending courses at dental meetings can also be very instructive and will assist one in keeping up to date.

Before Buying a Practice

❖   Before acquiring your own practice, it is better to work as an associate and gain knowledge and confidence in your skills. A patient feels insecure if he senses that the dentist is unsure about what he is doing. On the other hand, a patient is more at ease if he senses that the dentist is knowledgeable and secure in what he is doing.

❖   If you are still in dental school, an excellent way to acquire experience after you graduate is to work as a dentist in the Armed

Forces. It is a low stress environment (there is no pressure to generate an income) where you can concentrate more on quality and less in churning out fillings, such as can be the case in a practice that accepts capitation plans. Also, in the Armed Forces you will work with competent dentists who are willing and ready to teach you and help you with any difficulty that comes along.

❖   If you are considering acquiring a practice, a good location, generally, is one with major highways close by, for ease of access, and with plenty of free parking space available. The ease of access and free parking, though not fundamental for a successful practice, will nonetheless be a positive aspect for all involved: the patients, the staff, and you.

www.ingramcontent.com/pod-product-compliance
Lightning Source LLC
Chambersburg PA
CBHW081532220326
41598CB00036B/6412